REVE DISEASE NATURALLY

Natural Non-toxic Remedies and Forbidden Cures They Do Not Want You to Know About

By

Mike Cavalli

RB
Rossendale Books

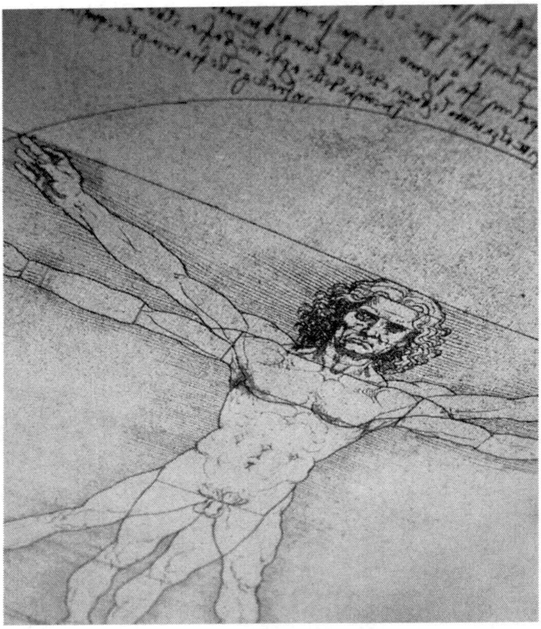

Photo of the Vitruvian Man
by Leonardo Da Vinci from 1492

Published by Lulu Enterprises Inc.
3101 Hillsborough Street
Suite 210
Raleigh, NC 27607-5436
United States of America

Published in paperback 2013

ISBN: 978-1-291-50071-4

CONTENTS

PREFACE

This book came into being over many unrelated but several serendipitous moments. When shopping I always had a curiosity as to what chemicals contaminated our food, health and consumer products and the possible long term damage they could inflict on our bodies. Even consumer goods such as TVs, cell phones and other wonderful goods I discovered had a ring of secrecy surrounding their compatibility to health and the human body.

In order to get a definitive answer and solve the puzzle once and for all, I had to keeping asking the question why, why, why, until no question was left to be answered.

Dogged determination and relentless pursuit through endless official, government, scientific and legal websites would not supply me with real information but arbitrary and quite often irrelevant information, the use of key words or *"search the site"* button would prove to be even more frustrating as it would often take me further away or back to the website that referred me to the site I was on. Speaking to real people, mostly functionaries proved futile and even more frustration than the virtual world simply because in order to get real information you need to speak to someone higher up the chain, and even then, at best they would be evasive and non-committal, *"you best look at The Food standards agency website or DEFRA"* and refer you back to a website!

I finally had my eureka moment, my reward for such audacity! I came across the legal framework that made it all perfectly clear as to why the law allows the corporate giants to be able to do and get away with their shenanigans, none so more than the cell phone industry!

De minimis non curat lex - The common law principle that judges will not address very minor breaches of the law - a loose translation is ***"the law will not concern itself with small matters".***

And so with so much valuable information at the helm, I reasoned *"how many people out there really know the truth about what they are eating, drinking, rubbing on their skin and sticking in their ear"?*

I was shocked to discover it was little or nothing at all simply because of the belief paradigm that government would protect us by outlawing anything that could be harmful, and so there would be no need to question the safety of our western lifestyle. We had become complacent in empowering ourselves and taking responsibility for our own health and our actions.

I had realized by now I had opened Pandora's Box! If so many people knew little about all of these issues, how much did they know about the various health care choices available to them?

A little knowledge can be dangerous, as a natural therapy consultant I would invite clients with certain conditions to consider the use Ozone therapy. *"Ozone! That's dangerous and illegal isn't it?"* But the truth is that while Ozone therapy equipment is not approved for medical use and therefore illegal for any professional to treat or cure disease with it, including Doctors, there is nothing in law to prevent any individual from using the equipment to treat or cure themselves.

I wanted to reach the masses with all this information, sharing the information ad hoc was too slow and laborious, I wanted to get the message out that with some personal consideration and paying a little closer attention to health and lifestyle choices, reversing disease naturally and that safely using approved protocols or forbidden cures was extremely plausible and as individuals the greatest thing we could do to regain and maintain good health is to take back control and responsibility for our own health, a very, very, powerful empowering protocol.

Drinking a tea at an airport lounge I got involved in conversation with a passer-by who looked somewhat tied and exhausted, we spoke a little about health issues and exchanged email addresses, three weeks later I received an email saying he took my advice on how to deal with long term fatigue and was now full of energy, radiant and most importantly had time for his family, he suggested that I should pen my work and *"get it out there",* and so my concluding serendipitous moment had arrived, the book came into being thanks to the perfect stranger.

REVERSING DISEASE NATURALLY

Natural Non-toxic Remedies and Forbidden Cures They Do Not Want You to Know About.

"Dance like nobody's watching; love like you've never been hurt; sing like nobody's listening and Live like it's heaven on earth."
Mark Twain

INTRODUCTION

Welcome and thank you for choosing this book on reversing disease naturally and equally as important a book that will guide you through the pitfalls that prevent you from retaining good health, keeping your body balanced and in harmony as natured intended.

I am excited to share with you the knowledge that is going to change your whole way of understanding how the body works, a paradigm shift in fact. I want to share with you research that I have made over a 20 year span and the new discoveries that I continue to learn each day. I am going to share with you the wisdom that has been handed down to me from medical scientists and medicine men.

You are about to embark on a journey, and along this path you will gather much information, and it is fair to presume that you may not be able to absorb all the information first time around. However the brain, this wonderfully complex yet perfect instrument, will almost certainly retain information that is important to you and nobody else. We are all unique. Our DNA, our RNA, fingerprints and irises are all unique. There are no two identical people and since we are unique and therefore special, what may be important to your healthcare needs may have no bearing whatsoever on me or anybody else: simply put - there is no one size fits all.

With your permission, I am going to empower you, giving you the confidence to take responsibility for your own health care needs, even when talking to your health care practitioner you will have the confidence to ask the appropriate questions, challenge his or her diagnosis and you will have the confidence to look for a second opinion, nothing is sacrosanct or carved in stone, nothing!

It is only fair therefore that I invite you to challenge information within this book. You may choose to agree with me on a certain subject, or you may say, well Mike, I understand the point you are making, but I am going to make some research of my own on this point, I need to know more about the subject. You could of course dismiss any part of this book as rubbish or that it simply does not apply to me! This is a good thing; this is empowerment, taking control of your own healthcare needs.

I would at this point also advise you not to be so bullish about this new found confidence, especially for those who have life-threatening bodily imbalances, please do take note of your practitioner's diagnosis, please do note the method he or she chooses to resolve the problem such as invasive or non-invasive surgery, the use of drugs, herbs or nutraceuticals, then you will prepared with valuable information to do your own research that will help you choose the methods best suited to you, your mind and body, there is no one size fits all.

UNDERSTANDING PAIN

Accepting the idea that there is no one size fits all should lead you to understand the sheer madness of walking into a drug store buying an over the counter product that reads something like; for mild pain, take one pill three times daily or for severe pain take three pills four times daily. Quackery, sheer quackery! How can these products define the severity of pain of individuals with surety?

There is a further problem we have to consider, those who suffer acute pain have developed a defence mechanism designed to trick the brain into believing that there is no pain, even though there are underlying physical symptoms. Simply put, this is called mind over matter.

Likewise, those labelled (sometimes inaccurately) hypochondriacs are equally capable of tricking the brain into sending a message of pain at the slightest twitch or cough, these people are commonly the "cup half empty" people, although it is worth noting that this also could be their own defence mechanism.

With this Understanding we can conclude that the product you are taking may either be rendered completely useless simply because the "real" level of pain you are experiencing is incompatible with the instructions on the label, worse still, some days or weeks down the line after taking too much of the OTC drug you may experience drug interactions, blood pressure changes, kidney function alteration, constipation and so on.

This problem does not only apply exclusively to pharmaceutical medicine, the same problems can occur with herbs, homeopathy, and nutraceutical medicine. For example, to continuously increase your dosage of vitamin C beyond the RDA in the belief that if you take enough of it will prevent you from getting a cold will only induce diarrhea, then you have reached saturation point, no matter how much Vitamin C you put into your body from here on in, it will probably do you more harm than good.

We need to be looking at this question of pain from a different perspective.

So what is pain? Unquestionably it is a local reaction to part of the body that is unbalanced, in other words, out of harmony with the self. Pain therefore could be conceived as a messenger, and it is this message (in the form of pain) that is presented to you because a localized bodily imbalance has been manifesting over a period of time to which you have not paid close enough attention to and as a final resort your body sends you this message: **PAIN! Now you will listen!**

But it does not have to be like this, if we were to slow down a little, still our minds, rest our bodies, breathe correctly, we could retrain ourselves to listen to our bodies joys, listen to her cries and understand once again what it is that she is asking from us to enjoy a balanced mind, body and soul.

Yoga, meditation, chi quong to name but a few can all help achieve this, whatever works for you. There is no one size fits all!

From this moment you have the opportunity to unlock the door to the part of the brain that has held you prisoner in the belief that:

"Only invasive surgery or chemo can cure me of my cancer" or that *"nothing can rid me of Arthritis it's just part of growing old"* or the best yet *"if alternative treatments worked, then my Doctor would be treating me with these methods"*.

FACT: Ophthalmic glasses do not cure poor or degenerative eyesight.
FACT: Imitrex does not cure migraine.
FACT: Asthma inhalers do not cure Asthma.
FACT: Analgesics do not cure Arthritis.
FACT: Prozac does not cure depression.

And we could continue endlessly citing drug after drug, and yet with just this information alone that we have shared thus far you can feel to be empowered.

THE LAW

Defining Medicine – The Codex - Food labelling law.

But before we take a look at how the body reverses disease naturally and the various proven protocols available to us today, we need to understand just a little about the law and natural health, for there is a very good reason why information is on a label and equally as important why, for example, missing on your favourite SEO or serialized electrolyte of oxygen is the information on how a powerful free radical scavenger this product is and if used correctly, subject to you are having enough repair tissue available in the body, can reverse even life threatening bodily imbalances, or why natures antibiotic, colloidal silver is sold only as a dietary supplement and not as medicine. For the same reasons when you purchase over the counter a bottle of DMSO (Dimethyl sulfoxide) it should read on the label "Sold as a solvent only". A product of the 60's, it was labelled "The silver bullet of medicine" but has since fallen foal of the regulatory authorities and has been granted only limited medical use to physicians; no medical claim is made anymore.

However the law in general stands like this. Should I squeeze some organic oranges put it in a bottle and sell it to you, that would be lawful, no problem there, however, should I sell that orange juice and say *"drink this yummy orange juice it will prevent you from getting scurvy,"* then I have broken the law on two counts. First, I have made a medical claim, I am not a Doctor, I am not authorized to make a medical claim, only Medical Doctors and those in the medical Profession can make such claim. Secondly, since I have made a medical claim, the orange juice has now become medicine and neither am I licenced to sell medicine. Similarly, should I sell you an organic brick and say *"go build a house",* this is legal, however, once again should I say to you, *"eat a little of this brick each day, it will cure your Arthritis"* then I have broken the law on three counts. The first two infringements we have just discussed and the third law I have now infringed is that I have sold you a product that has not been approved by the appropriate authority for curing Arthritis. The product has not gone through the often flawed, laborious and dated double blinded study, peer reviewed process, a process many forward thinking scientists and Doctors alike are asking the government to review.

The law is in a sense a good thing, it is designed to stop this type of quackery or snake oil sales, however it does have the tendency to tar all natural products with the same brush and therefore you will never see a medical claim printed on the carton of orange juice, neither will you see the supermarket making such claim on behalf of the orange juice manufacturer, why, because it is illegal for them also!

The most you will ever see on a label is *"can help you lose weight as part of a calorie controlled diet"* or *"calcium for healthy bones, speak to you Doctor about the benefits!*

The Codex Alimentarius

The Codex is probably the single most important body that affects our health. It is very complex and the official codex website will tax the patience even that of the most durable and persistent experts, it's a mega labyrinth that brings you around in circles.

I recommend for all information regarding The Codex you visit The Alliance for natural health's website at www.anh-europe.org/campaigns/codex

The Codex was formed 1963 and regularly reviews and amends its guidelines (Law) for member countries. Recent years has seen some of the most regressive guidelines being put in place and the worst is yet to come.

There is a positive list, an approved list of minerals and vitamins. Some of the minerals and vitamins not on the positive list includes several forms of natural Vitamin C and natural forms of folic acid, certain antioxidants, and a range of minerals including boron, vanadium & silicon, The positive list effectively bans 300 of the 420 forms of vitamins and minerals present in 5,000 products currently on the UK market.

Some substances on the positive list derives from genetically engineered crops, which means that since they are not natural, they are the property of presumably a corporation and therefore can be patented, but synthetic vitamin C and folic acid is not what you want in your body! The synthetic vitamin C along with the new lower RDA's will certainly prevent deficiency bodily imbalances such as scurvy. Vitamin D will prevent rickets, but they do not prevent complex chronic diseases which are on the increase due to micronutrient deficiency. In effect, the new guidelines will reduce the recommended daily allowance to a new safe level which will render them well below any therapeutic benefit.

Cancer clinics and Doctors using vitamin C in high intravenous doses will also be forbidden to use such high doses due to the new *"scientific risk assessments"* which will render that particular therapy null and void!

I highly recommend you see the film: *"We Become Silent - The Last Days of Health Freedom"*.

FOOD LABELLING LAWS

There are some basics you need to learn concerning labels, one could write a book alone on the subject, but the following examples should stand you in good stead when purchasing food products.

When is an organic fruit not an organic fruit?

A few weeks ago I went into a so-called health food store to buy some organic prunes and there they were on the shelf in big bold letters, ORGANIC PRUNES. Now if these prunes were truly organic then that is all the label should read, ORGANIC PRUNES, nothing more or nothing less, however as a force of habit I flip over the packet to see if there is "hidden" information, lo and behold, the label reads, organic prunes preserved in E621, (Monosodium Glutamate). As a consequence these prunes which may have started off life as organic have in fact been contaminated with the chemical E621 and made void the goodness of its organic value. In other words you would be eating an organic product with added chemicals. If organic is your choice, then it makes absolutely no sense in eating this product.

However, no law has been broken, the label clearly informs us that these prunes were grown organically, they have explained that it has been preserved with E621, but the producer has cunningly rendered this information in a place that you might not ordinarily look if you have not trained yourself to do so, or, although not a legal requirement, have they explained what is exactly E621.

Defining Meat: The flesh of an Animal

Meat is the flesh of an animal; well at least you thought it was!

Yet the law states that the minimum meat content of a pork sausage can be as low as only 42%. The equivalent figures for most other sausages are around 30%.

However, pork can contain up to 30% fat and 25% connective tissue and still be described as meat. The remaining ingredients include:

- "Rusk - to bulk and bind."
- Water- to hydrate the rusk (and because it's very cheap)
- Polyphosphates - to retain water.
- Soya - adds bulk and retains fat.
- Colours - (E100 - E180).
- Preservatives - (E210 - E239).
- Sulphites - preservatives to extend shelf life (E220 - E228).
- Nitrates - to give a pink colour and preserve (E249 - E252)
- Antioxidants - to prevent discolouration (E306 - E309, E320 and E321)
- Flavour enhancers - to enhance flavour (E620 - E640)

Mechanically Recovered Meat (known as MRM) can no longer be described as meat. The same goes for organs such as the heart and tongue. They can still be used but must be described separately on the label and do not count towards the minimum meat content.

Hence even should you buy a high quality sausage claiming to have 90% meat, remember that "90% meat content" may contain up to 30% fat and 25% connective tissue.

When is the country of origin not the country of origin?

As defined by FSA, "*the Country of origin is not defined in the law covering food labelling. However, when dealing with food from one country which is processed in another, the approach taken for food labelling is based on 'the place of last substantial change'. Broadly, this means that the last country in which a food is substantially changed is the country of origin*".[1]

In lay man's terms this means that you can for example import a pig that has been bred from Denmark, Ecuador or The USA, get it to England, then if you should make pork pies or Salami, then *"the last country in which a food is substantially changed is the country of origin."* Clearly this is substantial change and therefore it can be labelled as a British pig!

A Banger or a Sausage?

Another misconception we have developed is in the belief that a Banger is a sausage, colloquially we do call sausages bangers, but in real terms there is an enormous difference among the two. A pork Banger only has to contain 5% meat, the rest of the product does not have the same restrictions as a sausage, it can be filled pretty much with anything including some of the less savoury parts of the animal and often includes collagen, ligaments, tendons

A BANGER IS MOST DEFINITELY NOT A SAUSAGE!

Natural Flavours

When buying a product that reads *"with natural flavourings,"* or *"with natural spices,"* you might be forgiven for thinking that you are getting your favourite herbs and spices packed into one convenient package. Not so, the law has made provision for the big food manufacturing companies to process *"a flavouring substance (or flavouring substances) which is (or are) obtained, by physical, enzymatic or microbiological processes, from material of vegetable or animal origin which material is either raw or has been subjected to a process normally used in preparing food for human consumption and to no process other than one normally so used"* (Uk Definition of natural flavourings) In other words, the product only had to start out in nature from material of vegetable or animal origin (raw). What happens here in after is pretty much irrelevant.

But what you are not told is that the food regulation law of 1996 requires all ingredients (including food allergens) to be listed, in other words, if you were truly getting "natural" Rosemary, Thyme and Basil, then by law, the producer you would have to name them.

Remember, although something maybe natural it does not mean that it is safe or healthy!

COLOURINGS

A substance that has undergone 'selective extraction' for the prime function of colouring.

As with all government regulation, U.K. law regarding food labelling is a faux ami since it states that *"As with all other additives used in food, colours may only be used if they perform a useful purpose, are safe and do not mislead the consumer"*. Yet food colouring additives do mislead the consumer as they are used by manufacturers to serve several purposes. Most commonly to replace the products natural colours lost in processing, to make food appear more appetising or to mask the natural colour variants found in naturally grown produce. And although perhaps arguably acceptable, colourings can be used for decorative purposes on cakes for example.

It should be made clear and although at first glance may seem painfully obvious, you will see that it is not always so, colourings only add colour *"they are not substances that are normally consumed as foods by themselves or used as characteristic ingredients of foods."* [2]

When is an Ingredient a Colour?

In relation to food, a colour is not an ingredient if it has undergone 'selective extraction' for the prime function of colouring. For example, extracting the chlorophyll (the green colour) from dried spinach would be to perform a colouring function and these substances would not normally be consumed as foods alone, therefore would be labeled - chlorophylls (E140). If we simply take dried Spinach as used in producing pasta Verdi without extracting anything then its prime purpose is as you would expect an ingredient and would be labeled as such.

The law gets a little more complicated with liquids and as a consequence if you do not have the full picture on this part of the regulation, the rules are misleading. Here are two classic examples that describe perfectly the complicated law that the untrained and unsuspecting person will misinterpret.

Juices that are added to yogurts principally for colouring purposes and not added flavour are regarded as ingredients and would be labeled as such.

The colour caramel that is found in colas, leads you to believe that you are getting something natural, Caramel, but in fact you are buying a catalyst to disease!

Colour (caramel E150d) or Sulfite Ammonia Caramel

This has nothing to do with taste, it is merely a colouring.

The name suggests when you buy a soda the caramel you get is the natural unrefined brown sugar slowly melted over a warm heat to produce the Caramel. Not so. In fact what you are getting is Sulfite Ammonia Caramel. It is formulated by reacting sugar with both Ammonium and Sulfite compounds, the two by products of 2-methylimidazole and 4-methylimidazole have shown in numerous studies to be carcinogenic.[3] We will look at the hazards of soft carbonated drinks later on in the book.

MONOSODIUM GLUTOMATE OR NOT

The first point to understand about MSG is that it is a natural product, it is found in plants and Animals, it is an amino acid called L-glutamic acid, it is harmless as our body systematically breaks down through the digestive system the naturally bound glutamic acid.

We need this glutamic acid as it is a powerful neurotransmitter, is important for learning and memory and critical in the synergistic effect of two drugs, vitamins or herbs given simultaneously. However the free or processed glutamic acids is neurotoxic.

Many people are aware of the dangers of

this “excitotoxin”, and the big food manufacturing companies know it! For this reason they have “hidden” MSG in the food by renaming it, sometimes with a name quite appealing.

It is important to understand that should you consciously choose to avoid foods with MSG, then you need to understand the law on MSG since provision in the law can be confusing to both the untrained and trained.

In order to understand the labelling problem we need to look at Monosodium Glutamate from a different perspective.

Our rational mind tells us that if we read the label and MSG is not mentioned, then we are safe. Nothing could be further from the truth. MSG is just one of many flavour enhancers (E621) containing processed free glutamic acid.

Monopotassium Glutamate (E622), Glutamate, Glutamic Acid (E620), Gelatin (E441), Calcium Caseinate, hydrolysed vegetable protein, textured protein, Autolyzed plant protein, Hydrolyzed plant protein, Yeast extract, Glutamate, Yeast food or nutrient, Sodium Caseinate, and Autolyzed yeast are other flavour enhancers containing processed free glutamic acid, the very thing you are looking to avoid.

A label may say NO MSG or NO ADDED MSG but there are many hidden sources of MSG, these are very common in processed or convenience food, be sure to read the label

When Homemade means commercially prepared

When shopping and we cast our eye over a product that reads "homemade", we conjure up a picture of a simple domestic kitchen.

But according to the food standards agency website, [4] *"so as to avoid visual misrepresentation, factory-made foods should not be shown being made in small kitchens, farmhouses"* etc.

However provision in the law does once again accommodate the big food manufacturer to label their food homemade by; *"preparation of the recipe on the premises, from primary ingredients, in a way that reflects a typical domestic situation. This should not be achieved simply by the assembly of wholly pre-prepared elements, or simple reconstitution from dry base mixes, but must involve some degree of fundamental culinary preparation. As in domestic preparation, it would be legitimate for caterers to use partly-prepared ingredients that are available for domestic use; typical examples could include the use of pre-prepared raw pastry, bakery bread in desserts or stock cubes in sauces."*

If we look at the rule with more detail we find that the food manufacturing companies only have to *"reflect a typical domestic situation"* and involve *"some degree of fundamental culinary preparation"* plus the ruling can imply that homemade or domestic preparations can use partly prepared ingredients. This may or may not be the case, but the wording certainly tilts the balance in favour of the big commercial kitchen that is more likely to use partly prepared ingredients than the domestic situation.

Three issues need to be addressed. First, define “reflect”, what reflects for you may not reflect for me. There is no clear ruling in law, reflect is ambiguous and we can all therefore interpret the phrase differently and since it all comes down to opinion and interpretation this ruling can be exploited and is. Secondly, define “some degree”. Once again this is opinion and interpretation waiting to be exploited.

Thirdly, there is no provision in law for food manufacturing companies, (with reference to “homemade”) to use high quality ingredients. The rational mind tends to associate homemade food with wholeness and healthy ingredients. Caveat emptor, check the label for ingredients!

Fresh Fruit and vegetables

Once again we can be forgiven for thinking that "fresh" infers that the produce has been recently harvested, but the word "fresh" is now used generically to indicate only that the produce have not been processed (e.g. canned, pickled, preserved or frozen), it does not mean that they have been recently harvested!

Expressions such as "freshly cooked", "freshly prepared", "freshly baked", "freshly picked" should have no other connotation than the immediacy of the action being described. [5]

This leads us on to another problem, define immediacy? According to FSA guidelines; where such expressions are used, it is recommended they be accompanied with an indication of the date or time or period of when the action being described took place. I.E. *"freshly prepared this morning".* Packaging, storage and other supply chain processes that control "freshness" should not be described in terms that may imply that only a short period after harvesting or preparation has elapsed before sale if this is not the case. For example, a food that has been vacuum packed to retain its freshness should not be described as "freshly packed".[5]

In other words should you see a label describing produce as freshly packed or freshly picked, for it to meet the criteria of which you and I have come to understand the term, then it must indicate the immediacy, i.e. freshly picked this morning, freshly baked 2 hours ago, otherwise the producer has not met with the recommendation as laid out above, and this is only a guideline, they are not breaking the law should they choose to flout the ruling.

SULPHITES

Sulphiting agents (E220-24 and E226-28) are food additives that are widely used as preservatives in foods and beverages

Sulphites are regarded as one of the top food allergens and sufferers can experience a drop in blood pressure, rapid heartbeat, loss of consciousness swelling of the throat, hives, stomach pain, headaches, cough, fatigue, sinusitis, hyperactivity, memory loss, depression and difficulty in breathing, in extreme cases sulphites can bring on an anaphylactic shock closing the airways down completely resulting in death. Surprisingly, even The food Standards Agency admits, *"Prolonged high intakes of sulphites could cause stomach irritation, abdominal pains and vomiting. Ingestion of sulphites can cause bronchoconstriction or bronchospasm in some asthmatics."* [6]

It appears that more and more people are having problems with foodstuffs containing sulphites, so it's worth identifying the various names for Sulphites:

- E 220, E 221, E 222, E 223, E 224, E 225, E 226, E 227, E 228
- (European names) Potassium bisulphite/metabisulphite
- Sodium bisulphite
- Sodium dithionite
- Sodium metabisulphite
- Sodium sulphite
- Sulfur dioxide

- Sulphiting agents
- Sulphurous acid.

Those who are concerned by this relatively recent intolerance or those reasonably not wanting to introduce sulphites to their body will find the ruling on this subject quite complex and opaque.

The first problem to address before we recognize how to determine whether a food stuff contains sulphites is as you would expect is to understand the exceptions. Sulphites may be oxidised to sulphate, but the presence of sulphate is not routinely measured in sulphite food stuffs yet may affect to sulphur intake, in other words there is no requirement in law to mention that oxidisation can or has taken place (affecting total sulphur intake), or any harm it may cause you.

There are some foods that naturally contain sulphites such as garlic, grapes and onions, some dried fruits for example and it is reasonable that there is no requirement in law to mention this in a product.

The law only applies to ingredients that have been deliberately added and only when levels exceed 10mg/kg or in liquids 10mg/litre. Any levels under the threshold and there is no requirement for them to be mentioned on the label.

To make things more complicated manufacturers have several options of declaring (or masking the product) these totals declared by reference to the terms, *'sulphur dioxide' or 'sulphites', depending on the form of the ingredient added.* To confuse the public further manufactures can also use 'sulphites' (or 'sulfites') as a generic term for this ingredient. Manufacturers can also use the chemical name for a sulphite, therefore, in this case they can replace sulphur dioxide with sodium metabisulphite.

More people are becoming aware of the dangers of sulphites, but how many realize that sodium metabisulphite is a sulphite. A great way of masking the chemical!

One of the many nutritional deficiencies produced by this chemical is the destruction thiamine (Vitamin B1). Thiamine enhances circulation and the production of hydrochloric acid essential for digestion as well as creating good muscle tone of the intestines, stomach and heart. Smokers benefit from Thiamine as it tends to offset some of the damaged caused through tobacco smoke. Furthermore Thiamine is also a powerful antioxidant protecting us from the natural degenerative effects that comes with age. In extreme cases, and although rare in the so called developed world, one can develop Beriberi. Neurological symptoms include:

- Difficulty walking
- Loss of feeling (sensation) in hands and feet
- Loss of muscle function or paralysis of the lower legs
- Mental confusion/speech difficulties
- Pain
- Strange eye movements (nystagmus)
- Tingling
- Vomiting

Mothers breast feeding should pay

particular attention as Beriberi may occur in the milk due to Thiamine deficiency.

Asthma suffers can benefit from reducing or limiting their Sulphite intake. In a review back in 1985 entitled: Adverse reactions to sulphites.

The authors wrote, *"A level of sulfur dioxide as low as 1 part per million (ppm) may provoke airway obstruction in subjects with asthma."*[7]

So what is the safe upper limit of sulphites ingested for human consumption?

Impossible questions to answer since different products contain various Sulphites triggering various reactions.

The government has declared that Sulphites must be included on the label if they exceed 10mg/kg in foods or in liquids 10mg/litre. The question has to be asked how many hidden 10mg/kg and or 10mg/litre do we ingest on a daily basis before we burden our cleansing organs with this chemical to such an extent that the priority system that the body functions under can no longer cope!

An acceptable daily intake (ADI) of 0.7 mg/kg body weight/day has been set by the European Scientific Committee on Food (SCF).

In a study on the worst case scenario of The Acceptable Daily Intake (ADI) for sulphites, showed sulphite residues obtained from a combination of realistic meals high in sulphite-containing foods would lead to an intake of 23mg/day in children and 50mg/day in adults. [8]

HOW THE BODY HEALS ITSELF

Good science has shown that should we supply the body with the correct materials, then she is more than qualified to restore herself to a natural state of balance, harmony and wellbeing. Quite often and with patience, a safe detox program accompanied by supplying the correct nutrients and minerals to the body on a daily basis with good quality food or juicing can be sufficient to restore and maintain good health, sometimes we need outside help in the form of a protocol, or a non-invasive apparatus for relief from this temporary local trauma.

To speed up the healing process, much benefit can be gained by educating yourself with a little knowledge on the specific imbalance. For example as you age your bones lose calcium so you might want to consider foods rich in calcium such as Almonds, Beans, Broccoli, Halibut, Kale, Mustard greens, Orange, Tofu, to name but a few. With a little further research you will find adding vitamin D to your diet will help calcium absorption.

Poor blood circulation or Cold hands? Why not enjoy more foods with magnesium. Beans, nuts, peas, seeds, spinach, while whole unrefined grains are all good sources of magnesium. You will find after a period of time you will also gain more energy!

The book "Prescription for nutritional healing" is an excellent resource for assisting you in choosing the correct combinations.

Of course should your problem be somewhat problematic then you may want to do considerable research before you speak with your healthcare practitioner so that you can with confidence ask the appropriate questions.

Lesion

A wound or injury. A localized pathological change in a bodily organ or tissue. An infected or diseased patch of skin.

Let's take a look at what happens when we cut our finger, arguably one of simplest forms of local trauma.

As soon as the cut occurs your body immediately functions in the sympathetic mode, commonly known as the fight or flight mode. This is one of two modes, the other being the parasympathetic rest and digest or rest and recuperate mode.

The names are not important only the actions or more accurately the reactions.

As blood exits the wound, your body effectively says to itself, *"if I do not stem the flow of blood from the body then there is the risk of death"*. So the body constricts the blood vessels while blood platelets accumulate to form a clot, this process is called haemostasis or the inflammatory stage.

As the blood dries over the wound, a cause of oxygenation, a scab is formed sealing the wound preventing further loss of blood.

The skin now begins to heal, another process takes place called the proliferative phase, it is at this stage that the skin tissue begins the repair process. In the due course of time, when your body is ready, it will allow the scab to tear away from the finger revealing a perfectly healed lesion. It is this point, called the remodelling stage which can take place over months, even years, will continue to reduce scar tissue and replaces old damaged tissue with new, stronger and clean skin.

The finger has healed itself. We could of course assist in this process by putting pressure over the wound or even use a plaster to help prevent infection and stop blood leaving the finger or putting ice around the wound to speed up haemostasis but none of these functions repair or heal the body, they only assist in the body's natural ability to retain balance and harmony. Likewise a plaster cast for a broken leg or arm is merely an assistant, an aid to the best orthopaedic surgeon available, Corpus, the vessel of life!

Understanding the common cold and influenza

Common cold: A mild viral infection involving the nose and respiratory passages. Influenza: An acute contagious viral infection characterized by inflammation of the respiratory tract.

If you are one of those unfortunate people whom every time you come into contact with somebody with the flu, a cough or cold, and always go home with their symptoms then clearly your immune system is sluggish and your primary elimination and cleansing organs such as the kidney's, colon and liver are not doing their job efficiently due to a host of reasons, one of them certainly would be that your body is overloaded with toxins and or you have nutritional and mineral deficiencies. Somehow though, your perfectly engineered made by nature body finds a way of finding a solution to the problem, often in an approach that at first glance the rational mind recognises in the very least unwelcoming or unfavourable.

The common cold and influenza are just two shining examples of how we in the west have misinterpreted and consequently differ from the body's perception of this particular disharmony.

So you are around someone who has just sneezed and coughed all over you and through your nose, mouth, ears or skin go all his or her bugs and pathogens who find themselves the perfect home in your body where there is a comfortable temperature to exist and a good food source, let's take your stomach for example.

As the bugs and pathogens enter the stomach, mucus is formed to protect the stomach walls, as the bugs multiply more and more mucus is formed until eventually when the body can no longer contain the mucus, it throws it out, bugs and all through sneezing, runny eyes, phlegm, through the skin, passing water, and then the process starts all over again until all bugs, germs and pathogens are eliminated from the body. Your body is doing what it is designed to do!

We can hire the top 100 scientist and pay them trillions in research money to find a cure for the common cold, but we will never ever find a remedy for the common cold for the simple reason, the common cold is the remedy. Your body is doing what it is designed to do! The question we should be asking ourselves is not what pill or potion can I take to prevent a cold, but rather what is it that I am doing on a daily, weekly or monthly basis that allows with ease this kind of DIS-EASE within my body.

In years gone by the old traditional Doctor knew exactly the solution. Go to bed; wrap up warm, drink plenty of fluids. Why did he say that? Let's take a look.

By wrapping up warm the old Doc knew very well that the flu bug cannot live in very warm temperatures so by wrapping up warm the body induces a fever, (your body's natural defence mechanism) to a temperature above the normal body temperature of 98.6F and by doing so destroying the virus.

Drinking plenty of fluids would help

loosen the mucus enabling it to excrete the virus and rid them, drinking fluids also makes you want to use the toilet and by doing so you would eliminate these germs through urination.

A word of caution, complications and danger can occur if your body temperature induces a fever that stays around or above 103°F. Call your healthcare practitioner immediately!

Today though, somehow we have got it all back to front. The new Doctor comes along and says, here! Take this pill, it will reduce your fever; don't overdo it until you feel better, ciao!

The last thing we want to do is prevent your body's natural defence system from working, preventing a fever through medication is the perfect way to achieve this, resulting in more likely a prolonging of your misery.

Poor Vision

Myopia is the medical term for near sightedness. People with myopia see objects more clearly when they are close to the eye. Hyperopia, is also known as farsightedness. These individuals have difficulty with anything close-up while their general distance vision is not as bad.

The common misconception associated with age is that *"you are bound to need glasses, that's what happens"*. Yes it is true, to a degree there is a degenerative process that takes place with ageing but we can slow this process right down. One way of doing this would be to use the natural light of the day more often, avoiding the modern computer screens and TV's, digital advertising displays, flashing lights, neon lights, and the latest fade of electronic books all play their part in the downfall of our vision. Our eyes were simply not designed for this environment.

As soon as you hold the belief that as you age wearing ophthalmic glasses are natural, you put your eyes on a treadmill of deterioration. Ophthalmic glasses do not repair the eyes to restore perfect vision but merely use concave or convex lenses allowing light to hit the retina precisely allowing people with myopia or hyperopia to see as nature intended.

This does put us in a predicament as the end game is usually that of over a period of years, revisits to the optician for stronger and stronger lenses, more and more deterioration.

Now, let's look at the problem from our new perspective.

Why can I not see clearly without glasses? Why do I not have perfect or 20/20 vision? The answer is remarkably simple. It is all a question of light! To have perfect vision, the eye lens must send diverse angles of light rays or beams to a single pinpoint on the retina located at the back of the eye.

Should light from the lens not go directly to a single pinpoint it can cause the image to be unfocused, this is known as the blur circle and by squinting the eyes you effectively lock out these strayed light rays causing the problem allowing you to see clearer.

If you ever have watched somebody who wears reading glasses trying to read without them, they do exactly that, squint.

So how do we retrain our eyes to see unaided perfectly?

There are several exercises we can adopt. Many are freely available online and are almost all unconventional and they certainly get you to move your eye muscles again and most of you will feel the eye muscles pulling. Far too often in modern society through extended periods of computer use, reading tiny print in newspapers we have forgotten how to use our eyes correctly, we have become lazy and have become accustomed to very little eye movement. The healing process of restoring perfect vision will also be enhanced greatly by working in more natural light.

The Three Cups (for Focus)

Make sure the cups are at eye level!

Adjust your chair so that you are approximately 12 inches from a board or computer monitor with the two cups as seen in the picture above.

Hold a pen or any straight object vertically between the two circles approximately 1 inch from the screen keeping the top of the pen about the same level as the image.

Bring the pen towards your face (focusing at the top of the pen)

Something strange will happen, the two circles now give the impression of three circles. Stop moving the pen when all three circles appear to be same shape and proportion,

Move the pen and try staying focused on the centre circle; you may feel your eye muscles pulling. To achieve this it may take a day or so of practice, however it is not

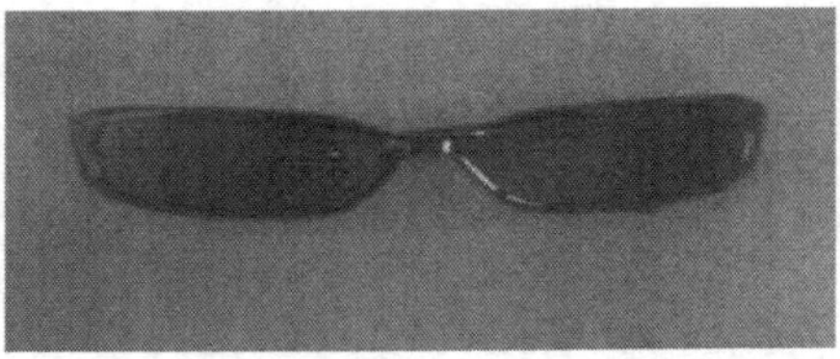

unusual achieve this on the first attempt.

As you maintain focus another phenomenon takes place, the circle will look three dimensional.

You should aim to do this exercise without the use of any instruments.

This is just one of many varied exercises available today. You can find many exercises online via youtube. But without doubt and certainly the least arduous, fun loving way to restore your eyes are with stenopeic glasses, (the Greek word meaning "little opening") otherwise known as pinhole glasses. They cost anywhere from £5.00 upwards. The difference in various prices mainly reflects design although the more expensive pinhole glasses are usually drilled with more precision, the difference is negligible.

These tiny precision drilled pinholes work much the same way as ophthalmic glasses but force these diverse angles of the light naturally to the back of the retina, they tend to block out the peripheral vision improving the sharpness of the image you are focused on.

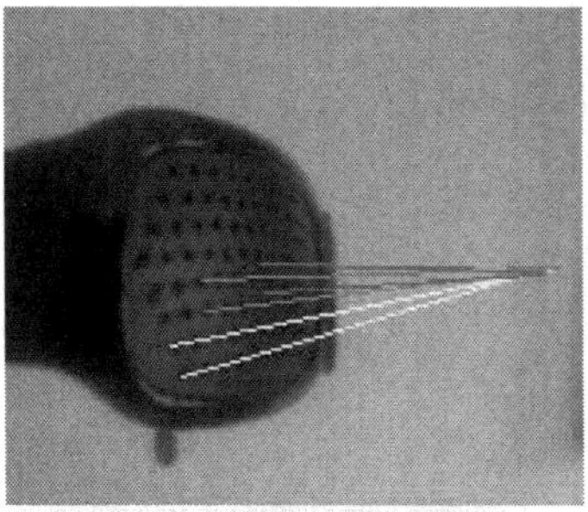

The various colours show how the angles of the pinhole glasses arrive at a single pinpoint

By applying these glasses to your everyday reading or when watching TV, your eye muscles will begin to move again, you will probably feel the eye muscles trying to pull themselves back into the way they have been accustomed to viewing objects. But this is a good thing, the movement retrains them, you develop eye muscle memory.

Designing your own structured plan for reading with the pinhole glasses or practicing eye exercises even for just 5 minutes a day is far better than the haphazard approach of as of where and when.

You cannot use the pinholes as an alternative to sunglasses; you will get a sharper vision though, but as a note of caution you should not look directly into the sun (after the end of sunrise and an hour before sunset) and since they do cut out peripheral vision you should also not wear them for driving.

HOW WE BECOME DISEASED

There only two ways our bodies become imbalanced. We either catch something such as a cold, flu, shingles and chicken pox and other communicative diseases or we develop an imbalance such as Arthritis, lower back pain, Cancer, Migraines, Tumours.

With the medical knowledge available to us to date, there are only four reasons how this happens.

1. Nutritional deficiencies - including vitamins, minerals & micronutrients
2. Toxicity – environmental and chemical
3. Electromagnetic chaos- A relatively new phenomenon
4. Emotional and physical stress

As we have come to understand with regards to medication there is no one size fits all. There can be a host of different reasons why for example somebody smoking 20 a day for 40 years does not contract lung cancer, yet another person who has not smoked does. Genetic makeup, the body's ability to detect and destroy "foreign cells" or the smoker may enjoy excellent and high quality nutrition off setting some of the many problems caused by smoking, while the non-smoker eats food with very little nutritional value.

The working environment is a factor greatly overlooked. A study printed in The international journal of Cancer reported: *Carcinogenic risks between hairdressers and personal users of hair dyes were evaluated by an IARC working group in 1992. There was consistent evidence from five of the six large cohort studies of an excess risk for cancer of the urinary bladder in male hairdressers and barbers.*[9]

It follows that there is no single reason for a particular imbalance to occur. So let's dispel a few myths:

Smoking is the cause of lung cancer. If that were true, everybody who smoked would develop cancer.

Coffee causes migraine. (likewise red

wine and cheese) Not true, if this was the case then everybody drinking coffee would have migraine.

Arthritis is what happens when you get old. Not true. There are many, many elderly people who live free of Arthritic pain, it's not luck, they are doing something right!

Looking at these problems from a fresh perspective, Ailing vision, bowel control, gum problems, diminishing concentration levels and so on do not have to be common place. As we age, unquestionably there is a natural degeneration process that takes place but we can slow them down or indeed prevent them.

It is important to understand that the body is more than capable of healing itself even from life threatening imbalances like cancer, provided we supply the body with good nutrition, we do eliminate all toxins from the body, reduce to a minimum the elctromagnetic chaos and most importantly make sure we are in a positive frame of mind as part of any protocol that we use in recovery of any imbalance, it is essential that you have exact information, happily in the final section I will document some of this best alternative treatments available, both home and clinical use.

All the above examples are secondary responses to local reactions and the answer for reversing disease and enjoying lasting good health lies in building a firm foundation to work from.

We should look at the four problems above as four simple rules.

1. To have always excellent nutrition.
2. Remove all toxins from our body.
3. Prevent or reduce to an absolute minimum Electromagnetic chaos.
4. Have a positive, creative, happy outlook on life (greatly disregarded as of any therapeutic benefit)

Is there a prime cause of disease? Almost certainly oxygen deficiency. But simply putting oxygen, real active oxygen (not air) into your body may be a waste of time unless we deal with the secondary causes.

The following examples will also reinforce understanding the consequences of oxygen deficiency, this single common denominator as the prime cause of disease.

NUTRITIONAL DEFICIENCIES

Chronic dehydration: When the body consistently has fewer fluids than it needs.

Chronic dehydration is one of the leading facilitators of disease, or to phrase it more accurately, chronic dehydration creates the perfect breeding ground for disease to manifest. It can cause inflammation which results in a variety of imbalances including: Arthritis, Asthma, Cancer, Diabetes, Heart Disease, the list goes on and on.

This mineral is greatly disregarded, it is the second most important element only to oxygen which without we can only survive for around five minutes. Without water we can only survive around 4-7 days depending on your size and how much water you had in you from the start of no intake, next comes food, we can last around 4-5 weeks, again depending on your size and body mass.

The body has no reserve water storage system; she relies entirely on water from an outside source. As a consequence she has built a defence mechanism to guard against dehydration. If a water crisis occurs, your body which works on a priority basis will transport water from a part of the body that she senses is not essential at the present time, sometimes known as "the now" to the locations she feels essential. Each and every one of us is individual, so no two responses to water shortage will be the same, similar maybe, but not the same!

Let's take a look at some imbalances that water dehydration is partly responsible for.

One problem dehydration causes lie within the duty of the cells. The cells which have hundreds of thousands of tiny pumps, if fully hydrated they will push out hydrogen peroxide which in turn neutralize (burn) the pathogens, grit and dirt that have accumulated around the knuckle joints causing swelling. The water then transports the debris to a disposal point, usually through urine or stools. But if there is insufficient water, your body could bypass delivering water to this point as it may have decided that water here is not a priority. Your body may have also considered that water held in the cartilage, (found between joints and used as a buffer) as a lubricant to prevent rubbing is currently unnecessary and should be taken and distributed to a more critical part of the body.

Arthritis

Arthritis: inflammation of a joint or joints.

For mild Arthritic sufferers, rehydration slowly and permanently can be sufficient to almost certainly reverse this process, reduce suffering and sometimes complete relief of symptoms is possible. Removing processed foods and red meat from your diet prevents inflammation thus relieving pain, swelling can also be reduced with one of the most powerful and natural nontoxic natural supplements, Boswellia Serrata.

Lower Back Pain

Lower back pain: is a common musculoskeletal disorder which affects the lumbar segment of the spine.

Relief from lower back pain can be found in rehydration. The disks, a form of rubbery cartilage between the vertebrae act as a buffer. To allow smooth movement of the vertebrae without experiencing pain, the disks need to be fully hydrated as their action is much like that of the shock absorbers on cars.

Water between disk and vertebrae work efficiently as a buffer once fully hydrated. Now, Imagine for one moment this cartilage as a small, partly deflated plastic or sponge ball resting between each vertebrae, there is insufficient water in the ball to form it's perfect round shape availing complete protection. As a consequence of the ball being able to be squashed out of its perfect shape, with certain movements the vertebrae touch, collide and scrape against each other. This is what is causing pain.

CANCER

Cancer: any malignant growth or tumour caused by abnormal and uncontrolled cell division.

Studies have shown that chronic water dehydration is a contributory factor in developing this imbalance.

1. Water carries oxygen through the body, cancer cells which have no antioxidant protection are destroyed by the oxygen.
2. Water dehydration allows toxic waste, pathogens and free radicals to remain and multiply in the body.
3. Water shortage raises acidity levels.
4. Water helps PH neutralize the body. It is very difficult for cancer to manifest in a PH neutral body.
5. Body Drought Causes stress. Stress is one biggest factor in facilitating disease.
6. Water shortage fails to transport vital minerals, vitamins and antioxidants vital for effective organ and immune function.
7. Most common cancers have all been linked to inflammation. And all inflammations have all been associated to a prolonged period of chronic dehydration.

Migraine

Migraine: A severe recurring headache.

Water shortage is without doubt one of the most important factors that should be taken into account when exploring possible causes of Migraine.

Water is a temperature regulator and when there is a water shortage it follows there will be a shortfall in the body's ability to regulate temperature. Numerous studies have been made on this subject with no conclusive outcome, but an overheated body can induce a headache, try staying outside in the summer months at midday. Thus the old age, "Mad dogs and Englishmen go out in the midday sun"

Tap water, generally regarded as dead water has many chemicals added to them for "purification," the two most known are Fluoride and chlorine and even more alarmingly talk of adding Lithium to the water supply. We will discuss these issues later on the book.

Soft Drinks

Soft drinks are generally carbonated drinks that are non-alcoholic. Carbonated soft drinks are also referred to as soda, soda pop, pop.

As with cigarettes, if we could go back to square one, then without any doubt the formula for soft drinks would today be banned, no question! They are simply too toxic and extremely carcinogenic and unless you know labelling laws you are left vulnerable and at the mercy of the various government agencies to protect you (and a pretty bad job they do of it too) from misinterpreting what we read on the label. Their job is to protect business by making sure that the products they produce do not give us disease or death in a timely manner that can be traced back to any one product, making it often impossible to prove a company's liability since disease can manifest over several years.

Food law, like other society's such as The Law society has its own interpretation of words and phrases different to common language found in the Oxford English Dictionary from which one can refer.

For example the word *assume* is defined as *"To take to or upon one's self; to take formally and demonstratively; sometimes, to appropriate or take unjustly"*. Yet in Law this term is defined *as "An agreement to continue performing duties under a contract or lease"*. Similarly the term moot is typically defined as *"Subject, or open, to argument or discussion; undecided; debatable; mooted"*, yet in law moot is defined as *"Not subject to a court ruling because the controversy has not actually arisen, or has ended"*.

Sports, science, health, all groups define words that best suits their society or organization and food labelling law is no different.

We "assume" what is written on the label is plain English, wrong! As I am about to point out you have been duped to the very grave detriment of your health!

In 2009 The UK consumed 6065 million litres of carbonated drinks (43% share of the soft drinks market) a rise of 2.2% on the previous year. This translates to an average of 98.3 litres consumed per person per year. The increased risk of disease grows with their profits. So let's break down the diseases available and understand exactly what the wording actually mean on the label of perhaps the most popular of drinks, Cola.

Typically the ingredients for cola are as follows:

- Carbonated water
- Sugar
- Colour (caramel E150d)
- Phosphoric acid
- Natural flavourings - (including caffeine)

The most controversial is carbonated water, controversial since in small amounts it appears to be harmless. Water is carbonated with Carbon dioxide, we expel CO2 from our lungs and we do not have any nutritional requirement for a daily infusion of CO2. Carbon dioxide does block Calcium absorption which makes the bones weak and brittle, thus we develop Osteoporosis.

Typically 330ml can of soda contains 35 grams of sugar, which is approximately equivalent to 6 teaspoons of sugar. Described commonly as a drug, an energy booster, toxic, even a silent killer, some journals report that an excess of this "drug" can lead up to 75 unpleasant metabolic changes. It causes obesity and Opioid Dependence. One 330ml can of cola will spike your blood sugar levels giving you an artificial high sending your body into shock excreting massive amounts of insulin which uses all the sugar available from the body and transports it to the cells. Your BSL comes crashing down leading to serious illnesses such as, heart and Kidney disease, stroke.

The Colour Caramel E150d, it is important to first understand that this is a colour and not a flavour, though the manufactures could use any other colour that is not associated with food but chooses not to, presumably since when reading the label we readily accept Caramel as a flavour. No doubt due to word association, we generally eat Caramel, we do not recognize Caramel as a colour unless you are an artist. This chemical is added to disguise the unsightly colours created by all the chemicals used to manufacture this killer drink. And this is where label deceptions come into play. The correct name for this laboratory made carcinogen is called Sulfite Ammonia Caramel. It is not Caramel as we have come to understand it, it is formulated by reacting sugar with both Ammonium and Sulfite compounds, the two by products of 2-methylimidazole and 4-methylimidazole are also found in some foods and tobacco smoke, it prohibits full development of organs and healthy cell growth, Inflammation of the epididymis (where the sperm is stored), tissue inflammation and studies showed that carcinogenic activity of 2-methylimidazole (2MI) was demonstrated in male and female rats and mice.[10]

A further study from Springer showed 4MI is carcinogenic inducing alveolar-bronchiolar adenoma and carcinoma in male and female mice. [11]

Phosphoric acid is used as a cleaner in various construction industries for removing mineral deposits, cementitious smears, and hard water stains, soak an old penny in some cola with Phosphoric acid for 30 minutes and see her gleam!

PA promotes low blood calcium level (hypocalcemia), PA promotes bone loss through calcium depletion[12], plus Phosphoric acid has an extraordinarily high PH value of around 2.8, and will rot the enamel from your teeth!

Information from The International safety data cards show that Phosphoric acid is corrosive to the eyes, the skin and the respiratory tract and most disturbingly corrosive on ingestion.

Caffeine is also added to the drink, it serves two purposes. First it is a diuretic, it encourages fluid loss through Urine, then you become dehydrated, since you are now hooked on sugar, (and soon caffeine) you reach for another cola! What you actually need is water! Caffeine, one of the most psychoactive substances in the world and is also very addictive, like any other drug consumers will soon need their daily fix, a very sinister move by the manufacturers adding this highly addictive drug to the drink as studies show that only 8% of the people in the study could recognize the taste of Caffeine.[13]

Those dependant on Caffeine will exhibit signs of increased alertness, inability to sleep and may experience dizziness, headaches and nausea followed by an almighty crash leading to depression and anxiety.

Have a Cola and you may not be smiling!

Acid Diet

An acidic pH can occur from, an acid forming diet, emotional stress, toxic overload, and/or immune reactions or any process that deprives the cells of oxygen and other nutrients.

Thus far we have discovered that chronic dehydration creates one of the perfect breeding grounds for disease to manifest.

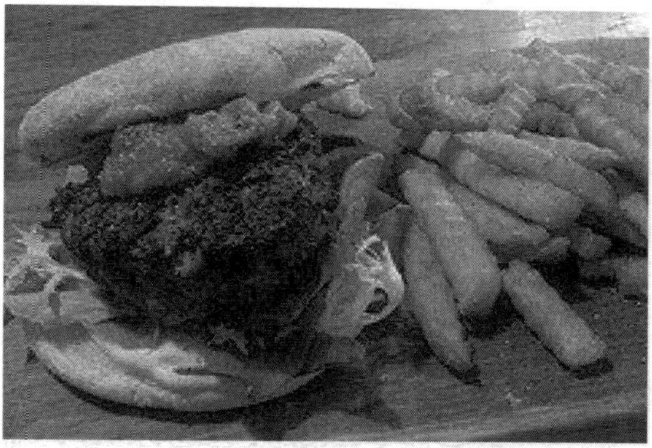

Photo by Annie Mole

A diet high in processed or refined foods are another means to which disease will readily manifest, even some vegetables are regarded as acidic forming. Corn has a PH value of anywhere between 5.5 to 7.0. Slightly acidic one must accept, surprisingly though, to some folk Tomatoes, regarded as a vegetable (botanically a fruit) is highly acidic with a PH value of 4.2 – 4.9. It is not so easy to define the PH value of meat as prior to slaughter the PH value is around 7.0 but increases as the body decomposes to around PH 5.4. Most soft drinks have a PH value of around 2.00 -4.00.

In order to maintain good bodily health, your body should be PH Neutral (PH7.4). Sadly, the western diet pays little creed to this observation and as a result we tend to eat highly acidic foods such as beef, goose, turkey, liver, veal, salami, rabbit, eel, halibut, herring, prawns, mussels, sardines, rosefish, salmon, peanuts, pistachios to name but a few.

Consumed frequently, these foods become disease magnets, breading grounds for disease to manifest. They can be inherently attributed to minor problems such as heart burn, now diagnosed as Acid Reflux Disease, or more serious problems such as heart disease, high blood pressure, raising the LDL cholesterol which in turn leads to hardening of the archeries, cancer from eating processed foods containing inorganic phosphates, a food additive found in meats, cheeses, beverages, and bakery products designed to increase water retention while improving food texture, once again the list is rather considerable!

Let us consider some popular diseases spawned from a highly acidic diet

Acidosis	An accumulation of acid in the body in which the body is unable to effectively eliminate or excrete through normal breathing or kidney function. Corrodes arteries, veins and heart tissues. Accelerates free radical damage. Promotes LDL cholesterol. Alters natural blood pressure levels. Macular degeneration. Can lead to MS. Inhibits cellular regeneration, inhibits oxygen reaching the cells, accelerates the risk of cell mutations (cancer)
Acne vulgaris	An inflammatory disease of the skin
Arthritis	Acute or chronic inflammation of a joint, often accompanied by pain and structural changes
Asthma	Shortness of breath, wheezing, COPD and emphysema and chronic

	bronchitis caused by inflaming the Bronchial tubes
Autoimmune diseases	Disorders in which the body's tissues are attacked by its own immune system. AIDS, ALS, (Lou Gehrig's disease) Cancer, Crohn's, MS
Chronic prostatitis	Inflammation of the prostate gland
Crohn's disease	Inflammatory disease of the intestines. It can affect the entire gastrointestinal tract from the anus through to the mouth. It can instigate Arthritis, Diarrhoea, inattentiveness, tiredness, weight loss, vomiting
Constipation	Causes a build-up of toxins as the colon is unable to excrete them, it can lead to colon cancer
Glomerulonephritis Hypersensitivity	Acute inflammation of the kidney. Prevents proper detoxification
Heartburn	A burning sensation in the chest or throat, difficulty in swallowing, sour or bitter taste, chronic coughing
Heart disease	Hardening of the arteries
Hypersensitivity	A detrimental reaction from the normal immune system. The responses may be damaging,

	uncomfortable, or occasionally fatal

We will also consider other factors that make the body acidic. Stress! Over a long period of time and quite rightly referred to as "The silent killer" stress will kill you. That is fact! Medical science though, is still not sure to this day why. A dynamic maybe the permanence of the fight or flight mode otherwise known as the sympathetic mode or possibly stress may elevate other problems such as LDL cholesterol, blood sugar and blood pressure levels to dangerously high levels and if left unchecked over a long period will get worse and can lead to a fatality.

Food preparation

An act of preparing foodstuffs for consumption.

Frying

There have been hundreds of books written on the disastrous effects frying and deep frying has on our health, so unless you have been living in a cave for the last 30 years or so there is no point in repeating the obvious, even if you are a newbie, you would have at least read or heard about the dangers of frying.

Frying destroys the antioxidants in oil and as a result oxidizes the oil. Oxidized oil becomes rancid and encourages the formation of radicals – free radicals cause cellular damage by, making the cell membranes stiff and inflexible which prohibit the transportation of vitamins and minerals necessary for good health. Fried oil also destroys nearly all nutrients and digestive enzymes required for good health, making your body work even harder to squeeze the remaining goodness out of the by now destroyed food.

Trans fats, an unnatural toxic chemical is the result of the process of hydrogenation. Hydrogenated oils, as you might expect are processed with Hydrogen gas to give the product a longer shelf life. Canola oil also known as Rapeseed oil is arguably the biggest culprit. The high temperature processing destroys much of the beneficial Omega 3 which in turn produces rancid odours converting some of it into trans fats. This triggers quiet an array of diseases including our old adversary heart disease by raising LDL cholesterol. Trans fats are named in being responsible for inflammation and blood clots which can lead to a stroke (or heart disease), impairs immune system function and increases in tumour necrosis. Some research also shows that just eating 4g of trans fats every day can lead to infertility in women.

And those that are fortunate enough to become pregnant often result in low birth weight.

Fast food addicts must take extra care as even if the restaurants they choose to eat in do not fry with hydrogenated products, deep frying foods at extremely high temperatures also creates trans fats.

A US study of Obstetrical & Gynecological from Lippincott Williams & Wilkins showed a 2% increase in energy intake from trans fatty acids was associated with a 23% increase in the incidence of Coronary Heart

Disease (CHD) **THAT IS JUST A 2% INCREASE**! The study also concluded that *"some results suggest that trans fatty acids may increase the risk of sudden cardiac death"*[14]

Once again, the food manufactures have realized that we are not buying into the health claims made by their marketing departments who pursue various cunning strategies to convince us, so do keep an eye out for the other hidden Hydrogenated products.

Look out for anything containing hydrogenated, partially hydrogenated oils, trans fats or shortened fats or oils.

Over and Undercooking Food

Here's a sobering thought. In USA The Centres for disease control and prevention in 1997 reported an outbreak of E coli due under-cooking food.

In a study prepared by Lancet, Heterocyclic amines formed in cooked meat and fish were carcinogenic in animal models and although the study suggests that if you remain within dietary guidelines for cooking and eating meat, the risk of developing cancer is minimal.

A Uruguayan Meat intake and chemicals study appears to disagree with the Lancet citing *"chemicals formed during the cooking process appears to be strong risk factors in human breast carcinogenesis"*. [15]

However a study presented in the Oxford Journals showed heterocyclic amines in cooked foods increases the risk of cancer by 80% for average consumption of meat. [16] In fact daily consumption of Bacon increases the risk of bladder cancer by 59%. [17]

But perhaps the most interesting findings were of a 1985 Swedish study which showed an increased risk of pancreatic cancer with continual consumption of fried and grilled meat which increased further with intake of margarine in contrast high intake butter which did not elevate the risk at all. In this study no known associations were found with coffee, artificial sweeteners or alcohol consumption, yet smoking increased the risk threefold. [18]

An additional drawback faced during the

cooking process is the release of acrylamides, (one of the many HCA's) found in over cooked meat but can be formed in some starchy food such as potatoes and cereal and although the exact temperature is not known when acrylamides are released, it is generally accepted that keeping the temperature below 120 degrees Celsius would prevent this neurotoxic chemical entering the blood stream. Symptoms of neurotoxicity arising from acrylamides are gradual, accumulating over many years and this is why it is almost impossible to identify the cause, but symptoms include cognitive problems, headaches, loss of memory, limb weakness and sexual dysfunction. They can even disturb neurons that process the information (signals) to the brain and nervous system. Parkinsons disease is the perfect example of a neurotoxicological imbalance.

So when cooking food bear in mind that frying or deep frying is positively the second worst method of preparing food only to microwaving as not only does this method destroy all nutrition and digestive enzymes, it also heats the food temperatures by up to 200%.

Refined Foods

Foods depleted of some or all vitamins, minerals and fiber.

Examples of refined foods include flour to produce biscuits, white bread, cakes and doughnuts. Processed meats such as Hot dogs and Salami are refined foods, likewise white sugar. A diet high in these foods almost certainly will lead to undernourishment and weight gain due to the enormous number of calories they contain. Often these products are bleached, copious amounts of salt is added and contain hidden nitrates.

It is quite common to find that after eating such a diet the "victim" often feels lethargic due to the body having to work extremely hard to squeeze out the precious little vitamins and minerals that remain. Your body works on a priority basis and blood will be directed to where it is needed the most, quite likely to the gut where a considerable amount of resource is required to help digest the acidic food, thus blood moves away from the brain making you sleepy. Consider also that refined foods cause the blood sugar levels to rise sharply giving you an artificial boost or high but send you crashing which results in low energy. To compensate, your body signals that more sugar is required resulting in craving more surgery foods thus a cycle of weight increase arises leading to addiction, obesity, heart disease and other complications.

The table below shows over many years some typical effects from a nutritional deficient diet.

Bones	Joints an bones ache - Brittle
Eyes	Cataracts – Bags or dark circles
Gums	Inflammation - Bleeding
Heart	Irregular beat - Enlargement
Legs	Tender calf muscles – Jolting reflexes
Mouth	Pale & sore tongue – Burning

	tongue – peeling & cracked lips
Muscles	Affects all skeletal muscle fibers, including respiratory muscles.
Nails	White spots – Ridges – soft or brittle nails
Skin	Dry, rough & scaly – Blocked hair follicles - Scurvy
Throat	Thyroid swelling

It should also be noted that Aches and pains - Arthritis - Weak bladder - Digestive problems – Lethargy – Osteoporosis are all signs of premature aging in younger people as a cause of nutritional deficiencies.

Salt

A colourless or white crystalline solid, chiefly sodium chloride, used extensively in ground or granulated form as a food seasoning and preservative.

Dr. Batmanghelidj, one of the most forward thinking doctors (now deceased) and author of the book, *Your Body's Many Cries For Water,* stated quite clearly that a salt free diet is utterly stupid.

Salt is found naturally in foods and is perfectly balanced by nature. According to The UK's food Standard Agency, the safe level of salt intake is 6 grams or 600 milligrams per day. Now providing you keep still, do not move, do not perspire, urinate, excrete or for that matter breathe, you will be doing fine. However for most of us, taking into consideration the above factors and depending on your body size and weight, you will need the recommended requirement of salt to maintain correct body function plus you may be required to take small additional amounts if you frequently run, or have a job that makes you perspire a great deal. Just check out those salt rings on your T- shirt!

The table below shows how detrimental the essential nutrient salt plays in a body's function.

Can weaken genetic defences if too much consumed in early life
Can lead to Heart disease
Can lead to Stroke

Causes high blood pressure with too much consumption
High intake can cause osteoporosis
High intake of salt can damage DNA (possible trigger for cancer)
Low salt intake can lead to acidity in the cells

This question of salt intake poses several questions. Many people believe that salt is sodium, well this is only a half truth, Salt is made up of 40% sodium and 60% Chloride. The regular table salt that most people use by definition, mass produced by the big commercial produces is most certainly not the salt that we require and depending on where you live in the world additives such as aluminium hydroxide or other anti-caking agents are introduced to give the product longer shelf life.

Aluminium hydroxide is also found in vaccine formulations whilst the Aluminium part of the chemical has been reported to be associated with Alzheimer's. It is used as a fire retardant and most importantly those undergoing kidney dialysis should use this with extreme caution as it can contribute to Aluminium toxicity. It can also neutralize acidity in the stomach; this can be both a good and a bad thing.

The high heating process in "manufacturing" table salt removes 82 of the 84 essential nutrients our body requires rendering this product pretty much redundant for our body's nutritional needs and can and is very often part of the process of disease formation.

Another factor we need to address is to know exactly the sodium we are ingesting. Many of the TV dinners contain excessive amounts of salt, they should indicate on the packet how much salt the product contains, but what of other off the shelf products. The table below [19] gives you some idea of salt intake from food.

PRODUCT	WEIGHT grams	SODIUM milligrams	Sodium grams
Cocoa powder	05	47.5	4.75

Cornflakes	30	333	33.3
Grilled bacon	40	500	50.0
Stilton cheese	25	287	28.7
Salami (3 slices)	90	1165	116.5
Omelette	100	1030	103.0
Salted butter	10	84	8.4
White bread (slice)	25	127	12.7

As you can see from the list it would not take long during the course of the day to send your daily salt requirement levels to go through the roof.

The solution to the salt question at first may seem to be extremely complicated, but in-fact the answer is rather straight forward, for most people it is often not necessary to spend endless amounts of time reading through the labels, you simply need to change your approach to the salt question, this does not mean that you will not be able to eat your favourite foods, on the contrary, with just a little bit of knowledge which I will share with you in the chapter on nutrition, you will find that in most cases, in consideration of the salt question, you will be able to eat all your favourite foods within reason.

It may require some balance, food such as Salami which is high in salt and nitrates which if consumed in large quantities and over a long period of time, will positively have adverse affects on your health. Remember also that through processing over 90% of the minerals we require are removed, plus the salt required for good health is not the natural organic salt which we will be considering in the chapter entitled Nutrition.

As a footnote, you ought to consider another anomaly in food labelling laws. Labels that claim the product is salt free can absolutely be not true! A food product can claim to be salt free providing there is less than 0.5g of fat per serving. Clearly therefore the product contains salt. The significance of this is when you are trying to watch your salt intake you can be taking in far more than you have calculated for. Salt intake of more than 0.5g per serving is regarded as high, but what if the product contains only 0.45g per serving, the manufacturer is not obliged to declare it, yet alone this product is pretty close to the high intake level, add that to other "undeclared" servings and you may end up wondering why, when you have been Conscientiousness about your salt intake, yet you have serious health problems!

Recently I was asked to make a report on the "benefits" and health risks of buying an economy frozen pizza. The findings will astound you and you will see that if you continue to eat these products which one can only loosely describe as food, then disease over a period of time is bound to manifest.

A Report on the health benefits and risks from frozen Cheese and ham Pizza

The purpose of this report is to not to determine whether you should be eating this product or not, rather to inform you of exactly what is in the product.

The information supplied is not conclusive in its findings as it may contradict official guide lines, even so many studies will back the findings.

This report should not be construed as medical advice.

The first question that needs to addressed is the place of manufacture and retail cost.

This product, a 12" pizza is produced and packed in Germany, shipped to England with a retail value of just £1.00. Taking into account all the costs involved should be an indicator of how nutritionally detrimental this product may be to the consumer.

The ingredients:

Wheat flour (Gluton) The flour produced from wheat has been bleached. Various bleaches are used but typically Nitrogen trichloride, It has the same effect as that of tear gas, but has never been used as such.

Gluton: Symptoms may include gas, bloating, loose or oily stools, constipation, fatigue, mood changes, depression and anxiety.

Rapeseed oil: Is poisonous to living things and is an excellent insect repellent. It is otherwise known as canola oil and is the cheapest oil to produce. It is a lubricant, agricultural fuel, used in soap, a synthetic rubber base and as an illuminate for colour pages in magazines. It is industrial oil. **IT IS NOT FOOD**

Yeast: Eating small amounts of yeast will do no harm.

Sugar: The product contains approximately 7g of sugar in the form of carbohydrates,

Food with 10g of sugars is regarded as high in sugar and those with less than 2g are low sugar foods.

Tomato sauce: The tomatoes used have more than likely been sprayed with pesticides and herbicides and have been reconstituted which means that the tomatoes have be reduced to a powder form and water added (which will contain chlorine and fluoride)

Potato starch is added to the tomato sauce which is a carbohydrate increasing your sugar intake.

Rice flour: Is used to thicken soups and stews, in this case it is added to the tomato sauce.

Paprika, garlic powder (sometimes containing stabilizers and chemicals) Oregano, pepper are added for flavour.

Colour Paprika extract E160c: It is important to understand that this is a manufactured colour and has nothing to do with taste. It is approved as safe by the EU it is banned in Australia as it may irritate the eyes and cause temporary blindness.

Chilli extract: It is probably the capsicum from the chilli that is being used although you should not touch your eyes with it as it will sting and give a burning sensation.

Black pepper oil: Has no known adverse effects on humans in small amounts. It is also used in aromatherapy oils and as a pesticide for repelling animals.

Vegetarian Mozzarella cheese: Suitable for Vegetarians as the enzymes used do not come from animal rennet (Stomach lining).

Reformed smoke flavour ham with added water:

Reformed ham is the tiny pieces of meat that is stuck to the tissue or bone and are removed mechanically and is reformed into a palatable shape. They are not cuts of good quality ham.

Smoked: Smoking a food product today is used usually for flavour rather than preservation. Smoked foods cause many problems if consumed in excess. They produce polycyclic aromatic compounds, well-known as a carcinogen. Smoked food is irritating for our digestive system and can be a contributory factor in to stomach and colon cancer, after many years of usual consuming.

Smoked Flavouring: The European Food Safety Authority (EFSA) says the flavourings used to give smoke flavour to meat, cheese or fish, may be toxic to humans. This is a flavouring and not the flavour produced from traditional smoking.

Sodium Nitrite: This is the preservative

that gives meat the pink colour rather than the natural decomposed grey colour. It also helps prevent bacterial infections. The Sodium content will also contribute to your sodium intake. The major concern regarding sodium nitrite is that it reacts with compounds called secondary amines to produce substances called nitrosamines. Nitrosamines, in turn, are potent carcinogens.

Dextrose: Also known as a corn sugar is a simple carbohydrate that rates very highly on the Glycaemic Index – It can give you a sugar rush and play havoc with your blood sugar levels. It is also used in energy drinks.

Stabilizers: These are used to give the product longer shelf life.

Salt: Salt is essential in our diet. Most probably the salt used will be table salt containing anti caking agents namely Aluminium hydroxide, AH is also found in vaccine formulations while the Aluminium part of the chemical has been reported to be associated with Alzheimer's. It is used as a fire retardant and most importantly those undergoing kidney dialysis should use this with extreme caution as it can contribute to Aluminium toxicity. It can also neutralize acidity in the stomach; this can be both a good and bad thing. The high heating process in "manufacturing" table salt removes 82 of the 84 essential nutrients our body requires rendering this product pretty much redundant for the purposes of our body's nutritional needs and can and is very often part of the process of disease formation.

UK government recommendations say that we should have 6mg of salt per day. This product weighs 370g per serving and contains 1.3 g of salt per 100g. This is equal to 4.80g of salt; almost at the guideline limit. Consumers should also note the hidden salt in the smoking process of the ham.

Water: Most probably the water used is tap water and depending on where you live may contain fluoride, a neurotoxin and almost certainly chlorine, a highly toxic gas.

Diphosphates: Used to prevent

discoloration of food. Excessive use can lead to demineralization of bones and can lead to fractures.

Triphosphates: Sodium triphosphate, Pentasodium triphosphate, Pentapotassium triphosphate are used in food to retain moisture. There are no known side effects when used in foods. Although high concentrations of phosphates may disturb several metabolic processes as phosphate plays an important role in general metabolism namely kidney function.

Antioxidant Sodium Ascorbate: (E301) Other names include Acid sodium salt, Ascorbicin, Ascorbin, Cebitate, Cenolate, Monosodium Ascorbate. These will more than likely be manufactured in a lab and not the natural product extracted from vitamin C. It is used as a preservative namely in cured meats. The sodium in this chemical should be added to your daily Sodium intake. Excessive amounts can lead to high blood pressure.

Report Conclusion:

From a nutritional perspective this product offers very little as it seems to be overloaded with arguably quite harmful preservatives, colourings, flavourings and stabilizers. The meat is of the poorest quality (reformed). The body would have to work very hard to squeeze the nutrition, minerals and vitamins from this product.

The high quantity of salt associated with this product can pose a health risk when you consider food consumed from other sources during the course of the day.

There is a considerable amount of sugar in this product which is also heading towards the recommended daily allowance.

It is difficult to determine exactly how much salt and sugar are in the product as some of the sugar and salt is hidden or found naturally in the food. Cooked ham although a protein contains carbohydrates, a complex sugar.

Long term consumption of this product alone would increase the probability of disease.

This report is for educational and debate purposes only and should not be construed as medical advice.

If you have any questions about ingredients in any food product you should consult a nutritionist or your health care practitioner.

NUTRITION

The process of nourishing or being nourished, especially the process by which a living organism assimilates food and uses it for growth and for replacement of tissues.

In the last chapter we looked at the endless array of means to become nutritionally deficient, so let's address these issues and see how we can continue to enjoy our favourite foods and drinks, but rather than harm us, give us the minerals and nutrients that our body requires.

Nutritional Drinks

The exciting news is that there is an endless array of nutritional and enjoyable fluids on the market to satisfy everybody's needs and desires even die hard soda fans can still enjoy their favourite cola that causes less damage, the downside of all this is that you may have to shop outside the big commercial superstore and look at a specialist health food store.

Water

Water remains our second most valued element only to oxygen. We have no reserve system so our body relies on us to supply sufficient quantities.

Consider this. Depending on the size of the person, we on average lose through breathing alone approximately one quart (USA) or 33 fluid ounces in Europe, (about four cups of water) each day.

As a rule of thumb, and there are no hard and fast rules to how much water you should consume, but the general census of opinion by the experts are that you should drink approximately half your body weight in ounces. So if you weigh 100 llbs then you should drink 50 ounces of water (that's almost 1.5 litres), if you perspire or work out you will need more.

Quality of water is important; we have discussed the problems from drinking tap water, thus it should be avoided if at all possible. Drinking mineral or spring water typically contain and will help to contribute to your daily required intake of:

1. Bicarbonate – to help balance acid alkaline fluctuations.

2. Calcium – get some of you required daily calcium from water.

3. Magnesium – Cell energy production and bone growth / maintenance

4. Sodium – Helps transport nutrients and debris to required parts.

5. Potassium - Controls blood pressure and can help to prevent strokes

Bottled mineral or spring water also contain between two – seven ppm of oxygen, while distilled water contains between seven- ten ppm of oxygen. But undoubtably the best water to drink is ozonated water from a natural non-carbonated source. This water contains up to 50ppm of oxygen and consumed twice or three times a day will not only contribute to your daily required water consumption, but the active oxygen will destroy any pathogens and bugs in your body since like cancer they cannot live in an oxygen rich environment!

Distilled Water

Distilled water produced by reverse osmosis (RO) still holds much debate. There are two schools of thought. One school says that the water is dead, reverse osmosis removes everything minerals and all.

The other agrees, but makes the claim that it is absolutely pure! The solution, should you choose to drink distilled water is to take a good variety of plant derived minerals as opposed to rock based. Once your body is fully hydrated using good quality water and remains hydrated, we begin to witness the body healing many man made imbalances:

- Arthritis suffers find their pain is eased or in some milder cases disappear totally.
- Asthma sufferers find that they too can breathe easier without wheezing.
- Lower back pain disappears.
- Cognitive abilities improve – clarity of mind.
- Encourages easy passage of waste through the digestive system and helps soften stools. (Reduced risk of colon

cancer)

- Helps you lose weight by suppressing appetite.
- Kidney function becomes more efficient.
- Liver function becomes more efficient.
- Muscles become less brittle and more elastic!
- Rids the body of toxins.
- Reduces cholesterol as it is soluble in water.
- Regulates body temperature.
- Relaxes muscle tension to allow freer flow of blood.
- Transports nutrients more efficiently to their required place.

It should be noted that if you increase your water intake you will through urination loose some of the salt that your body requires to function correctly, this applies also to increased perspiration so it may be necessary to add a pinch of Salt to your water to keep your salt levels to around 6g per day.

Organic Soda

Organic sodas will contain colourings and flavourings, that is just the way it is but the damage caused to the body if consumed in excess is considerably less. The table below highlights some typical ingredients in organic Soda's.

Cola	Sparkling water, Organic agave syrup, Organic lemon juice from concentrate (2%), Barley malt extract, Lemon flavouring, Cola flavouring.
Lemonade	Sparkling water, Organic agave syrup, Organic apple juice from concentrate (15%), Organic cloudy lemon juice from concentrate (4%), Lemon flavouring.
Root beer	Sparkling filtered water,, organic evaporated cane juice, organic root beer flavour, organic lemon juice concentrate, organic vanilla extract.

You can also juice your own drinks; lemon squash, cranberry juice, apple juice, pear juice, prune juice, plum juice to name but a few. To extract the maximum nutrition from these wonderfully refreshing drinks you should juice them and immediately drink them as the enzymes will start to break down immediately on juicing.

Juice And Drink Is The Golden Rule!

Below are a variety of drinks readily available in health stores that perhaps you will be unable to juice as importing laws may require transported goods across the seas may need to be irradiated.

Aloe Vera	A detoxifier, colon cleanser, aids healthy digestion, natural immune Support, maintains healthy skin through collagen and elastin repair, contains vitamins A, B1, B2, B6, B12, C, E, Folic Acid and Niacin, contains 19 amino acids, and 7 essential amino acids, for the gums it has natural anti-bacterial and anti-microbial actions.
Blueberry juice	Prevents urinary tract infections, protects against cancer and reduce rapid tumour growth, protects against heart disease.
Coconut juice	High in electrolytes and minerals that help to re-hydrate the body Contains lauric acid. An antimicrobial, anti-bacterial, anti-fungal and anti-protozoal. Helps to carry nutrients and oxygen to the blood cells and has been shown to raise the metabolism and help clean the digestive tract. Helps ease suffering of gastritis.

	Cools the body and helps retain correct body temperature.
Goji juice	Supports the health of all the cells in your body, supports the immune system and cardiovascular health, boosts energy levels and stamina, fights free-radical damage.
Noni juice	Helps maintain healthy skin, assists in clearing acne, can relieve constipation and stomach ache, helps prevent hair loss and has cancer fighting properties.
Passion fruit	A digestive stimulant, contains high amount of fibre, high in vitamin A, antioxidants found in passion fruit have been found to inhibit the growth of cancer cells.
Alfalfa	A rich source of dietary fibre and chlorophyll, calcium, phosphorus, chlorine, magnesium, potassium, sodium, silicon and Vitamins A, B, C, D, E, K and G, can assist Arthritis patients, can assist high blood pressure and disorders of the heart, stomach, and respiratory system.
Camomile	A relaxant so it can assist with insomnia and other sleep disorders, relaxes muscles, can help with menstrual cramps, stomach flu, and ulcers.
Green tea	Reduces the risk of esophageal cancer, lowers *total* cholesterol levels, can help with rheumatoid arthritis, cardiovascular disease,

	increases metabolism so can assist in weight loss programs.
Peppermint	Can treat irritable bowel syndrome, eases nausea and vomiting, controls flatulence, dissolves gallstones, fights bad breath, clears congestion and coughs (related to colds and allergies), can control mild asthma and is a stress buster.
Yerba	A diuretic, strengthens heartbeat, breaks down stored glycogen in the liver, breaks down fats, stimulates the central nervous system.

A PH Neutral Diet

A solution or substance that is neither acidic nor alkaline.

When the body is PH neutral it is very difficult for disease to manifest, so it makes sense to maintain a PH neutral body, this can be done fairly easily as foods are generally categorized as alkaline or acidic forming.

As a guide you can assume that most grains (but not all) are acid-forming while vegetable and fruit juices are highly alkaline. A PH neutral body is considered to be around 7.4

There are many debates over a healthy

diet, how much protein, how much carbs and roughage, the answer once again lies in our individual unique needs. Traditional guide lines suggest that in adulthood we need less protein, it is suggested by doing so you can reduce your chances of coronary heart disease, this may be true, but these guide lines refer to meat, poultry, dairy, eggs and fish. But there are other nutritious forms of complete proteins (a complete protein contains all nine essential amino acids) that will reduce further the risk of heart disease. Houmous, Soya beans, Tofu, Tempeh and Quinoa, to name but a few. I am not advocating you switch to a vegetarian diet but you can get all the protein your body requires and reduce the risk of heart disease by reducing your animal protein intake and replace it with proteins suitable for vegetarians.

Many times the question is asked. What percentage of carbs/proteins and fats should my diet consist of? And once again the answer is inconclusive. Certainly if you have the body imbalance called cancer eating a diet high in surgery foods or carbohydrates is not a good idea as it serves to feed the cancer. Arthritics should reduce or cut down their intake of red meats particularly refined meats such as bacon and sausages as they have proven to cause inflammation, and replace it albeit temporarily with complete proteins vegetarian style! Some schools suggest a forty - thirty – thirty ratio. This may be fine, but what if you are doing a job that requires a lot of energy!

Certainly as we age protein becomes even more important to maintain muscles, prevent hair falling out and help maintain healthy nails.

Until such times as you are able to judge your own body's requirements, those without internet should visit the local library and take a photocopy of the government food pyramid chart while those with internet can download the government food pyramid.

Good Food Preparation

Tastes, looks and smells delicious, is fresh, wholesome and pure and has nutritional value.

When addressing food preparation, there is in fact only one way to prepare food and that is to consume food as nature intended! This effectively rules out for the most part cooking and if we keep to the strictest of nature's rules, then, we should eat food raw. However we are not going to do this so we need to address this issue and define the best way of enjoying our food without suddenly sending the body into shock.

As discussed previously, frying, boiling and microwaving destroy nearly all the enzymes we require to maintain good health so this is not an option. So how can we prepare our vegetables without killing off the goodness that they promote.

Vegetables

Fortunately for us science has discovered that should we heat our vegetables in a temperature that does not exceed 104F (40C) then we slow down dramatically the progression of enzyme damage, therefore your vegetables should not be soggy since even cooking them below 104F for long periods of time will result in loss of enzymes. Minerals and vitamins are also lost but this does vary on the type of food you are cooking. One benefit of eating as nature intended is that it aids digestion.

It is certainly a good idea to have the body used to the idea of eating partially raw food, salads are a good example, but we can also include or add as a side dish, grated carrots and cabbage, thinly sliced beets and chicory, the list is quite exhaustive.

Other means of cooking that reduce enzyme damage are steaming and baking. Rice can be steamed as well as vegetables and you do not need to go without chips (fries) if this is your preferred choice. Once again you simply have to change you habit. You can either bake them or should you have a big enough griller, grill them, this way you will in the very least prevent the damage caused by frying or deep frying.

Even if you like the taste of the oil you do not have to feel left out, simply brush over the chips with your favourite cooking oil and you have pretty much got what you normally have but with more nutrients, enzymes and minerals without the disease promoting frying method!

As a footnote, you can help yourself further by making sure that you are fully hydrated a full thirty minutes before eating and that you desist from drinking thirty minutes prior to consumption. Once you begin to eat you can continue drinking again. Digestion is greatly eased as the water helps produce adequate stomach acid to aid digestion.

Chewing food into smaller parts creates saliva which in turn aids digestion by allowing the body to use less energy and assimilate more easily the food into the nutrients, minerals and vitamins. By doing so you also prevent damage to the oesophagus as smaller particles will not force and scrape the food down the tube.

Oil And Vinegar

Listed below can be eaten raw or dressing be added to them. By making some simple changes your body will receive a powerful boost in its defence against disease.

Flaxseed oil	Rich in essential fatty acids – aids digestion – reduces inflammation - used to prevent and treat heart disease – lowers cholesterol.
Krill oil	Effective in reducing Arthritis – helps lower cholesterol – can help reduce symptoms of premenstrual syndrome - contains astaxanthin a powerful antioxidant.
Hemp oil	An anti-inflammatory - contains omega-3 therefore reducing risk of heart disease – contains the rare protein globule edestins (to the globulin found in blood plasma.) – Helps prevent Eczema-like skin eruptions.
Olive oil	Can help lower blood pressure – a powerful antioxidant – can assist getting rid of gall stones – reduces the risk of cancer – reduces risk of heart disease (oleic acid) – supports bone health.
Sesame oil **(The queen of oils)**	A natural antibacterial - Cell growth regulator – Nourishes the scalp to help prevent dandruff - Helps keep joints flexible - Inhibits the growth of malignant melanoma – Helps maintain good

	cholesterol.
Walnut oil	Improves blood circulation - Lowers risk of heart disease – Helps maintain correct hormone levels - Improves skin –Anti aging effect.

To get the maximum benefit of these oils you should not use them for heating. As a guide the best oils will come in dark glass bottles (to prevent sunlight damage) and not plastic bottles as it is well documented that the thalites from the plastic leach into the oils contaminating them with harmful toxins.

You should also look out for cold pressed oils, better still single pressed cold oil.

Vinegar

Vinegar has been used throughout the ages for its various healing qualities applied both topically and for consumption. It acts as a flush for the kidneys and used as a tenderizer and an antibacterial on food.

The liver is the only organ in the body to be able to regenerate itself, but those with liver conditions or weakened liver should realize that taking too much vinegar can lead to cirrhosis (hardening of the liver) leading to further complications. Also if your body is in an acidic condition then consuming more vinegar will only make your condition worse, so while the benefits of vinegar out way the downside, as with all things, air on the side of caution.

There is but only one brand of vinegar that can have a dramatic effect on our health and that is Apple Cider vinegar with the mother.

It is essential that the vinegar contains the mother. The Mother is a natural phenomena as a result of the manufacturing process; it is friendly bacteria and an essential part of the goodness in vinegar.

APPLE CIDER VINEGAR WITH THE MOTHER

A powerful antibacterial	Athletes foot – Candida – other fungal infections.
Anti-inflammatory	Assists with Arthritis – Asthma – Eczema and other inflammatory imbalances.
Enzymes	Aids digestion -Contains natural enzymes, vitamins and minerals

	and is also rich in antioxidants.
Beta carotene	Assists in repairing damage caused by free radicals.
Blood sugar levels	Can help maintain correct BSL's – aids in the prevention of diabetes thus preventing further complications.
Calcium	Can work synergistically to extract calcium from other foods.
Pectin	Fibre – reduces cholesterol – flushes colon thus helps prevent colon cancer.
Potassium	Regulates blood pressure - glucose to glycogen and maintain healthy kidneys, heart and liver – prevents calcification of the soft tissues – promote proper bone health.
Toxins	Assists the body to break down toxins – flushes the liver & kidneys.

Unrefined Foods

An unrefined food or other substance is in its natural state and has not been processed.

In the previous chapter we spoke about refined foods so the table below shows some examples of unrefined foods. You will not be surprised to discover that once you start looking you will easily know the difference; you will understand that you can in fact eat your favourite foods but merely have to change some bad habits.

Unrefined Foods	
Beans	Azuki - black soybeans – chickpeas - kidney beans - lima beans – lentils - Tofu.
Roots	Burdock – carrots – parsnip - radish - Celery - chives – cucumber - green beans - green peas - sprouts.
Sweeteners	Brown sugar (whole grain) - maple syrup - stevia – xylitol. **In fact unrefined sugars are in endless supply.**
Vegetables	Broccoli - Brussels sprouts - buttercup squash - butternut squash – cabbage - cauliflower - greens – kale –leeks – onion - parsley - pumpkin red cabbage - turnips - watercress.
Whole grains	Barley – buckwheat - bulgur – brown rice - cornmeal - corn on the cob couscous – millet – Quinoa - rye – Spelt - whole oats - Whole wheat berries - whole grain bread (prepared from unrefined grain).

Vitamins v Whole Food Supplements

Vitamins are organic components in food that are needed in very small amounts for growth and for maintaining good health. Whole food supplements are a preparation intended to supplement the diet and provide nutrients, such as vitamins, minerals, fibre, fatty acids, or amino acids, that may be missing in a diet.

There is much debate over which is better, vitamins or whole food supplements. In an ideal world, if we ate as nature intended then we would have no need for either, and even if we are the most conscientious consumer, the modern day agricultural methods of growing and harvesting food has left the food chain chronically deficient in nutrients and minerals that we so badly require, therefore we need to supplement our diet with one or the other. Supplement is the key word. Mistakenly, good intended people have allowed their rational to believe that by taking supplements of any description plugs the nutritionally deficient holes. These products are supplements only, designed to supplement and not replace what-ever is deficient in your body. As by now you will not be surprised to discover pumping yourself with vitamins, minerals, enzymes and other supplements will without doubt lead to other complications. Balance is the key as an August 10 2007 study in the journal "Cell" revealed that the oxidative stress caused by excessive antioxidants may lead to heart disease. [20]

As discussed briefly earlier in this book, if vitamins are your route to get the maximum benefit then they need to work synergistically promoting the absorption of other vitamins and minerals. For example if you suffer from Arthritis then a blend of calcium, magnesium and vitamin D is a product available, missing one of these elements may not do the job and you will have wasted your money. Likewise for suffers of Carpel tunnel, a blend of Coenzyme Q10 and coenzyme A is often recommended, one without the other may be useless.

However, if you do not have a specific problem then whole food supplements are the direction to go, and there are many available, just look at this list of powerful superfoods, immune boosters and antioxidants found in one particular brand of whole food supplements. **Feed your body!**

Acerola Extract	A powerful antioxidant - astringent – acts as a diuretic - prevents diabetes – promotes healthy heart function – a liver stimulant - rich in vitamins and minerals – reduces inflammation.
Apple fruit	Rich in vitamins A B1 B2 B3 B5 B6 B9 Vitamin C – contains (amongst others) calcium – iron magnesium – potassium and zinc – rich in fibre – contains tannin which helps prevent gum disease - helps maintain correct level of estrogen for women – can help reduce cholesterol.
Broccoli Sprouts	Helps prevent cancer – stomach disorders and peptic ulcers – reduces heart disease risk- help prevents macular degeneration – helps prevent oxidative stress caused by diabetes.
Cauliflower Sprout	An anti-inflammatory -Helps prevent all types of cancer – contains vitamin C, K and manganese and omega-3 fatty acids - contains antioxidants that lowers the risk of oxidative stress in the cells - provides cardiovascular and digestive support – protects the stomach lining.
Collards	An excellent source of vitamins B6 and C – carotenes – chlorophyll and manganese – a source of fibre - minerals

	include iron, copper, and calcium.
Cordyceps	Boost lung capacity - combats weakness and fatigue - strengthens the immune system – strengthens cardiovascular function - increase energy- and stamina levels.
Kale	Rich in nutrients: Antioxidant- anti-inflammatory and cancer prevention properties – cholesterol lowering – regulates, thus promotes safe detox.
Kale Sprout	A good sources of dietary fibre and B vitamins – high in folate and iron.
Maitake Mushroom	Builds immunity – fights cancer – regulates blood sugar.
Nettle	A diuretic - can reduce allergy symptoms – helps reduce swelling of haemorrhoids.
Parsley	Helps prevent tumour formation – prevents oxygen damage to cells – increases antioxidant capacity of the blood – vitamin A & C - A source of folic acid – protects against Arthritis .
Pure Beet Juice	Blood pressure regulator – aids digestion – helps prevent circulatory disorders - can prevent dry skin, acne & dandruff - lowers cholesterol - helps prevent the formation of cancerous tumors – a powerful detoxifier - increases stamina.
Pure Carrot Juice	Vitamin A B E – helps maintain healthy bones - eyes– liver – teeth– nails – helps prevent cancer – helps liver function.
Pure Spirulina	A beta carotene food with full spectrum of carotenoids – anti aging – promotes cell regeneration - proven to fight

	malnutrition - stimulates beneficial flora - promote healthy digestion –promotes good bowel movement – helps eliminate mercury and other deadly toxins - increases stamina - helps build muscle mass – can curb hunger – contains copper, chromium, iron, manganese, selenium, zinc, - reduces bad cholesterol - Support the Liver and Kidneys - **Truly a super food!**
Reishi Mushroom Mycelia	Anti-stress properties – enhances liver function – inhibits neurological disorders – anti cancer and tumour properties - fights cholesterol.
Shiitake Mushroom Mycelia	Anti-tumour properties - enhances the immune system especially against bacterial infection – protects against anti-viral activity – Can help stop tooth decay.
Spinach	Anti-inflammatory- anti cancer – contains vitamin A, B2, B6, C, E, K, calcium, copper, folate, iron, magnesium, manganese, niacin, potassium , selenium, Zinc – an excellent source of protein – promotes a healthy heart – protects against eye disease – prevents cognitive decline.
Tomato Juice	Contains lycopene, a cancer fighter - Vitamin C – potassium – stimulates blood circulation – lowers blood pressure – improves appetite and digestion.
Wild Bilberry	Packed with antioxidants – anti-inflammatory - helps prevent cellulite - wrinkles – promotes healthy collagen –

	helps prevent varicose veins and heals bruising – detoxifies the intestines – protects against colon cancer – can prevent urinary tract infection – improves night time vision.
Wild Blueberry	One of the highest cellular antioxidants – Fights oxidative stress - can reverse short term memory loss- promotes healthy aging – promotes motor skills – an anti-inflammatory - protects against cancer – protects against strokes – improves night vision.
Wild Lingonberry	A rich source of fibre-sugar, vitamin A, B, C - calcium, magnesium, phosphorus, sodium and potassium - a rich source of Omega-3 – anti-inflammatory - protects against cancer – acts as a natural diuretic – Assists with liver ailments – gastritis - hypertony and gastric ulcer – neutralizes toxins- aids digestion – helps to prevent infection - lowers cholesterol – balances blood pressure.
Pure Chlorella	A powerful detoxifier for heavy metals and pesticides – cleanses theblood, bowel, and liver – contains digestive enzymes - improves digestive system - fights cancer – helps balance the bodies PH – can normalize blood sugar and blood pressure levels.
Organic Rice Maltodextrin	One of many carbohydrate sources in meat replacing products – allows the body to process food more easily – helps prevent over eating.
Organic Amla	An antioxidant -high in vitamin C –

fruit	enhances food absorption – promotes healthier hair - a natural temperature regulator – a detoxifier - promotes and improves cognitive abilities and muscle tone – provides support for the urinary tract – regulates stomach acid – anti aging.

Probiotics

A microorganism introduced into the body for its beneficial qualities.

These microorganisms or dietary supplements can help replace some of the goodness that food preparation has destroyed, they are somewhat already present in a normal digestive system so it matters not whether you are a vitamin or whole food type of person everyone benefits from probiotics! The benefits of these microorganisms in promoting good health include:

- Aids digestion and can help with gastritis
- Assisting immune function
- Breaks sown hydrocarbons making food easier to assimilate and digest
- Cleanses the intestinal tract
- Helps kill parasites and viruses, thus

promoting good health

- Normalizes bowel movement
- Prevents yeast infection
- Provides antigens that fight disease
- Provides support to eliminate toxins
- Provides antibodies

Digestive Enzymes

The breaking down food in the course of digestion.

Once again we have to address the missing links in our food chain and the culprits are food preparation and modern day farming methods. Both of these processes, unless you eat raw foods and grow your own food on soil as nature intended is going to leave you short of digestive enzymes that we so badly require.

If we do not digest our food properly then some of it can remain in the stomach where it will rot which in turns causes its own little chain reaction of turning this somewhat putrid substance into a wonderful source of nourishment for pathogens and bugs. Worse still what does not get eaten eventually will turn toxic and cause a build-up in the colon, and unless these toxins are not removed they will seep out of the colon and transported around the body.

Another good reason for a regular colon cleanse!

The enzymes provide us with a multitude of benefits and without them life ceases to exist. They provide us with cellular energy and also help repair damaged tissue and organs. They also help break down the food more effectively providing us with more nutrients and as a consequence can reduce hunger. What a way to lose weight!

The digestive enzymes contain four essential elements to support us.

- Amylase digests carbohydrates
- Lipase digests fats and oils
- Maltase digests sugars and fats
- Protease digests protein.

As we age, we lose the ability to produce enzymes and this is why you can no longer eat or tolerate your once favourite foods, so supplementation is essential to maintain good health, eating some raw foods will certainly give a big boost in making sure you get your share of enzymes, but some foods such as carrots are hard to digest, in these cases you should grate the food and eat immediately.

There are some tell-tale signs that you may be lacking in enzymes, you have experienced them already but have not connected it with enzyme shortage. Allergies, bloating, constipation, heart burn, supressed immune function and ulcers may be due to this imbalance.

Eating when you are tired or fatigued will almost certainly mean your body will have to work harder to process the food, another reason to take digestive enzymes, and of course eating slowly, chewing the food breaking it down into smaller pieces with or without enzymes will make for smoother digestion absolutely!

Sodium

A common metallic element of the alkali group, in nature always occurring combined, as in common salt.

There are many beneficial products on the market now many of them can be found in the high street mega supermarkets so you do not even have to go out of your way, just remember that you want a product preferably with nothing added neither taking away, as in table salt where the process of manufacturing rends it pretty toxic.

Salt, naturally plays a very important role in maintaining good health, it is essential also to maintain a Salt/ potassium diet.

Salt intake remains outside the cells and in between the tissues and offers many essential roles in the maintenance of health:

- Absorption of food particles through the intestinal tract
- Correct salt intake prevents osteoporosis
- Clearing of the lungs of mucus and phlegm
- Helps transport nutrients and oxygen through the body
- Helps nerve pulses work effectively
- Maintains water balance in the cells
- Prevents muscle cramps
- Required for proper potassium/salt

balance
- Required to make bicarbonate and stomach acid for digestion

Whilst Potassium, an ionic salt found naturally in fruits and vegetables and in sea water plays a crucial role in maintaining healthy cells. ***Note that around 98% of the Potassium remains in the cells.*** The list below shows the health benefits:

- A major role in reducing blood pressure
- Assists in ridding the lungs of carbon dioxide (breathing out)
- Converts glucose into muscle fuel (glycogen)
- Essential to maintain correct nerve and muscle function
- Good for acid/alkali balance regulation
- Maintains kidney function
- Regulates all cell activity
- Regulates the heart beat
- Required for normal fluid balance with sodium

It is crucial therefore to have a balanced Salt/Potassium diet. As a guideline it is accepted that the body requires five times more potassium than it does salt and as you might expect it is difficult, almost impossible to give typical examples as our body's needs are all different. In the previous chapter we spoke about salt intake and you should refer to this chapter. But for examples of food sources with various degrees of Potassium, see the table below.

High	**Medium**	**Low**
Apricots	Apples	Asparagus
Avocado	Broccoli	Blackberries
Bananas	Carrots	Cabbage
Dates	Celery	Cooked Rhubarb
Figs	Mango	Grapes
Prunes	Plums	Onions
Artichokes		Radishes
Potatoes		
Spinach		

Some of these various "healthy" salts available may have to be bought in specialist shops.

Herbal salt – Typically produced with sea salt. Different manufactures produce herbal salts with various herbs, but typically you can expect to find; basil, celery leaves, chive, garlic, kelp, leek, rosemary & thyme included in the product.

Himalayan salt – Pinkish crystals that contain all the elements our body requires and can be used to make Sole (solay), a natural heavy metal detoxifier

Pan Salt – Contains around 40% less sodium in the salt and contains lysine, magnesium and Potassium. (Other salts often do not contain these)

Sea Salt – Probably the safest bet if you are new to the various salts available and their numerous benefits. Commonly used in gourmet cooking and is produced by evaporation rather than industrial processing, thus leaving most of the essential elements intact for proper body function. Due to its high mineral content, including iron, sulphur and magnesium (but is a poor source of Iodine) sea salts have more flavour than toxic table salt, thus you may need less than your usual quantity in cooking.

TOXINS

A poisonous substance or substances that can cause disease.

Thus far we have discussed the various poisons and solutions in our food chain, so now let's look at what is described in the stores quite absurdly as healthcare and sanitation. Absurd simply because the unbelievable amount of harmful chemicals found in these products simply render them null and void for health benefit, yes they may make you smell fresh and keep your hair in place, but this daily build up toxins has indisputably led to very serious health conditions. Once again I would like to point to the fact that often the build-up of toxins in the body is so slow taking place over many years that no one product can be brought to book! They are numerous so we will only take a look at some "popular" toxins

Alcohol

A colourless volatile flammable liquid, C2H5OH, that is the intoxicating constituent of wine, beer, spirits, and other drinks, and is also used as an industrial solvent and as fuel.

It is common knowledge that in moderation certain types of good quality wines and beers can have some therapeutic use. It has been well documented also that whiskey with a drop of warm water has a calming affect for people in shock. The general opinion in the use of Alcohol discovered from the numerous scientific studies suggest that in moderation Alcohol does no harm to the body.

There are however some important issues that we need to consider, and as you might expect, quality is of our primary concern.

A typical example would be; should you buy a 75cl bottle of wine that has come from South America, you can expect to pay around £3.99 per bottle upwards. The excise duty imposed by The UK treasury is approximately £2.00 per 75cl. The product needs to be transported half way around the world, bottled and distributed. The supplier needs to make a profit as do the merchants selling the goods. The question we need to ask ourselves is, what exactly am I drinking that has been labelled wine? Common sense tells us therefore that cheap wine may not be beneficial to us at all!

We know that during the fermentation process that Sulphites are produced, daily consumption of alcohol may increase your Sulphite intake way above the Acceptable daily intake (ADI) contributing to problems previously discussed.

Safe levels of Alcohol for men are considered to be 21 units of alcohol per week but to be consumed in quantity's no more than three units per day. Women should consume no more than 14 units of alcohol per week, again with no more than three units per day.

One reason for the safety levels can be found in ethyl alcohol (or ethanol) the main chemical compound found in Beers, wine, Bourbon, Whiskey and others, it is toxic, in fact all Alcohol is toxic to the body. Ethanol is used in the manufacture of varnishes and perfumes and is often used as a solvent in the manufacture of paints.

One of the effects Ethanol has on the human body is that inhibits human bone cell proliferation (production of new tissue) and is generally accepted as one factor in heart disease and cirrhosis of the liver, an important cleansing organ for the blood.

Expectant Mothers should pay particular attention to Alcohol consumption as studies have shown that the Ethanol content in alcoholic consumption can produce various toxic and potential toxic responses in fetal tissues which can lead to spontaneous abortion as a result of hypoxia. Furthermore a 2003 study concluded that *"Consumption of five or more units alcohol per week* (a large glass of red wine has approximately 3 units) *and 375 mg or more caffeine per day (One cup of coffee may contain between (0.1 g to .15 g of caffeine) during pregnancy may increase the risk of spontaneous abortion"* Expectant mothers should also note that caffeine intake may be increased through other drinks, sodas 12gm's, instant coffee 55gm's, and white Tea 15gm's.

Ironically the study also showed that women who smoked 10–19 cigarettes and 20 or more cigarettes per day did not have significantly increased odds ratio for having spontaneous abortions, after adjusting for other risk factors.[21]

The effects on the liver due to alcohol abuse are devastating and well documented, the question we need to ask ourselves therefor is, expectant mothers aside, how much alcohol on a daily basis will we need to consume before we do damage. The answer as you may have deduced by now is somewhat impossible to answer since everybody is different, we are all unique, our Body mass index differ from person to person, our, shape and, size, the level of optimization of our immune system and cleansing organs all vary, so there can only be a guide, common sense and taking responsibility for your own body is what is required here.

But as guide, a twenty five year study in 2007 entitled: Alcohol Consumption and Alcoholic Liver Disease: Evidence of a Threshold Level of Effects of Ethanol, concluded that *"no significant increase in the incidence of features of alcoholic liver disease (ALD) could be related to all-year daily intake of ethanol below 40g (40g equals 1.1 liter of beer, 0.44 liter of wine, and 0.11 liter of spirits. In contrast, similar duration of daily intake between 40 and 80g (mean 61.6g) increased the risk of all but fibrotic liver lesions of ALD significantly and may thus represent a potential threshold level that significantly increases the risk of alcohol-related liver damage."*[22]

The table below highlights some of dangers of excessive alcohol consumption.

Alcoholism	An addiction or dependence
Average volume of consumption	Mouth and Oropharyngeal cancer; Oesophageal cancer; Liver cancer; Breast

	cancer; Unipolar major depression; Epilepsy; Hypertensive disease; Hemorrhagic stroke; Cirrhosis of the Liver
Altitude	Can cause breathing problems on high altitudes. Brain A psychoactive drug. A depressant (not a stimulant) Causes mood changes. Can increase risk of Dementia loss of inhibition
Bones	Inhibits human bone cell proliferation
Diuretic	Forces water from the body
Fetes	Can induce Spontaneous abortion Can affect nutritional intake Hypoxia Reduction of oxygen supply to a

	tissue below physiological levels
Hands, feet & speech	loss of motor coordination
Injury - intentional injuries	Unintentional and were found to depend on patterns of drinking in addition to average volume of alcohol consumption
Old age	Can increase risk of Dementia
Underage drinking	Associated with brain damage and neurocognitive deficits. Impaired intellectual development may continue into adulthood

Aspartame – An Excitotoxin

A derivative of aspartic acid and phenylalanine.

I have resisted placing the dangers Aspartame in the nutritional deficiencies part of the book even though it is used as a sweetener in drinks and foods. It is branded under the names of Equal, NutraSweet and Spoonful and now Amino Sweet. This highly toxic chemical produced arguably by a company with one of the most checkered history is responsible for over 75% of reported adverse food reactions. Anxiety attacks, breathing difficulties depression, dizziness, irritability, heart palpitations, muscle spasms and memory loss to name but a few. In more severe cases seizures and death pursue!

Aspartame is made from 40% Aspartic acid, 50% Phenylalanine and 10% Methanol

Aspartic Acid - Phenylalanine

Aspartic acid is a glutamic acid and is found naturally in protein rich foods, it is natural and safe and many of the these protein chains are joined, but Phenylalanine and aspartic acid are singular, they are only amino acids being introduced to the body. When the Aspartic acid is not bound it enters the central nervous system at an alarmingly high volume "exciting" the neurons so vigorously that it kills the cell! It is this reaction that is responsible for some of the adverse reactions such as headaches and mental confusion and cognitive difficulties.

Methanol

Methanol or wood Alcohol is flammable and poisonous and as you might imagine is a chemical you want to avoid consuming, but worse still, when Methanol is cooled it creates a by-product which we all know of, formaldehyde, or embalming fluid! Formaldehyde is also found in cigarette smoke, fuel-burning appliances and wood products. Industrially it is used as a disinfectant, germicide and fungicide. Even The National Cancer Institute in a study declared a link between formaldehyde exposure and death from cancers typically of the blood and lymphatic system found in workers at formaldehyde plants.[23]

A Cesare Maltoni Cancer Research Centre study in 2005 concluded that "*Aspartame is a multipotential carcinogenic agent even at low daily doses of 20/mg/kg of body weight."*[24]

1996 An American Association of Neuropathologists revealed an exceedingly high brain tumour rate in rats feed with Aspartame.[25]

Headache: The Journal of Head and Face Pain, in a 1989 study concluded that aspartame may be an important dietary trigger of headache in some people.[26]

The evidence against Aspartame is overwhelming, it is best avoided even if you are trying to lose weight, and there is no conclusive evidence to suggest that it does!

Antiperspirants

Before we become acquainted with the problems faced when using Antiperspirants, let us first address why we need antiperspirants in the first place. We are toxic! Clear and simple! And antiperspirants actually contribute to the increase in toxicity levels in the body resulting in odour (BO). We should not use them and once again at the risk of repeating myself, if we lived and delivered nutrition to our body's, and lived how nature intended then we would not have a need for antiperspirants, period! It is essential for good health to allow the toxins to leave the body, antiperspirants do not allow this, in fact they have the opposite effect, and they force toxins to stay in the body. Part of the function of perspiration is the process of ridding the body of toxins. Typically antiperspirants prevent sweating by forming layer of Aluminium over the pores of the skin under the arm pit. This evidently does cause local toxicity and since the toxins have been transported to the armpit for disposal they now find their exit blocked and travel back down the lymph glands and pass to the lymph nodes in the breasts. Due to the daily build-up, the toxins remain in this area and are one of the prime suspects in breast cancer for women.[27]

So let's look at what you can expect from a typical can of antiperspirant.

Aluminium Chlorohydrate.

A salt used to block the pores.

Reacts with or corrodes active metals, including structural metals as Aluminium and iron
May cause severe burns to skin and eyes
Toxic if inhaled, ingested or skin contact. May cause severe injury or death. http://www.chemicalbook.com/ChemicalProductProperty_EN_CB7396252.htm

Aluminium zirconium tetrachlorohydrex

A salt used to block the pores.

Aluminium has been established as a neurotoxin
Can cause contact dermatitis
Is dangerous if inhaled
Possible association with Alzheimer's disease

Hydrogenated Castor Oil – Stearyl alcohol - Triglyceride-

Provides structure and stabilization.

No known adverse reactions except in

lethal doses

Propellants

Butane

Can cause frostbite on contact with eyes
Can cause frostbite on contact with skin
May cause effects on the central nervous system

Isobutane

Can cause frostbite on contact with skin
The substance may cause effects on the cardiovascular system resulting in impaired functions and respiratory failure. Exposure at high level may result in death.

Propane

Can cause frostbite on contact with eyes
Can cause frostbite on contact with skin
On inhalation can cause Drowsiness and unconsciousness

Aluminium

The concern for Aluminium in products is

growing, rightly so it is linked to dementia and by reducing the use of Aluminium you reduce your chances of developing Alzheimer's considerably.

Let us not forget Aluminium production is an industry and as a consequence must turn in a profit each year and will look to find new ways of introducing this toxic product to as many products it possibly can.

Below are some of the products found to contain Aluminium.

Some of the common symptoms to aluminium toxicity are: Cognitive problems - Dementia - Breast cancer – Dermatitis – Osteoporosis - Psychological disorders - Rash

Healthcare	Food & Drink
Antiperspirants	Baking powder (not baking soda)
Body lotions and creams	Beer and soda cans
Cosmetics	Cutlery
Hair conditioners	Foil

Medicine	Pickles, cheese and baking soda. (Sodium Aluminium phosphate)
Shampoo	Pickled vegetables
soap	Processed foods (dietary aluminium)
Suntan lotion	Pots and pans
	Water

Unfortunately it is a case of reading and understanding the label whether it is a healthcare product, food or cutlery it makes no difference to your body! Many manufactures hide the Aluminium content by renaming it relying on consumer ignorance. Some products use a compound called Aluminium Silicoaluminate. Other products, antiperspirants for example may claim that they use no Aluminium Chlorohydrate but may substitute it with Alum, claiming that it is not Aluminium.

To summarise; Aluminium is a product best avoided especially in later years and we require no biological need for it. Reducing your intake of this chemical can seriously enhance your wellbeing as it can free your immune system and cleansing organs to concentrate on other important tasks. We have no back up, our immune system works on a priority basis only!

Chlorine

A highly irritating, greenish-yellow gaseous halogen, capable of combining with nearly all other elements.

Chlorine is added to water as a purification treatment, but once again this chemical can do us much harm and has a sinister and chequered history.

Chlorine was first used in World War 1 in the form of chlorine bombs.

The troops would toss the bombs over to the enemy dug in the deep trenches which would produce a yellowish cloud, at first it thought to be a smoke screen to allow the advancing troops cover. However as this yellow gas moved closer to the defending troops, they at first experienced coughing, then respiratory problems and finally death, such is the power of chlorine.

Some of the dangers of Chlorine are listed below:

- It contains trihalomethanes, a known

carcinogen

- Aggravates Asthma
- Is a strong irritant
- It destroys much of the intestinal flora that is needed to aid good digestion

The World Health Organization (WHO) has recommended that chlorination should be maximized at five parts per million (ppm) depending on where you live, the ppm will vary. A general guide is you can expect 1 ppm from tap water. That is just 1 part per million. It is minuet, yet the damage to the respiratory system and the ability to cause degenerative disease over a period of time is undeniable.

Taiwan like the USA and UK has been chlorinating water and a study showed that there is *"a positive association between consumption of chlorinating drinking water and cancer of the rectum, lung, bladder, and kidney."*

Conclusion: *"MX is a potent carcinogen in both male and female rats, and it causes tumours at doses that are not overtly toxic to rats."*[28]

"The risk estimations carried out indicated that each year 1 of the 5 million Ankara residents could get cancer from the daily intake of water, mainly because of exposure to chloroform through oral ingestion."[29]

Fluoride

A compound of fluorine - A by product of the fertilizer and aluminium industry.

Fluoride categorized as a part II poison in UK which means it must be kept separate from food products and sold sealed.

There are many different types of fluoride, the two that concern us are Sodium fluoride found in toothpaste and Hexafluorosilicic acid found in water. But this is only a half truth.

Sodium Fluoride

Until recently Sodium Fluoride was the only ingredient used in rat poison, it was used first in the Gulags and then in the concentration camps as it was found to kept the prisoners docile, as a consequence most antidepressants will have some form of fluoride as one of their active ingredients.

Countries all over the world vary the amount of fluoride permissible in toothpaste, but as a general rule it ranges from 100 – 1500 parts per million (PPM). Some toothpaste do not even declare fluoride content.

In the Uk, toothpaste with sodium fluoride comes with a warning simply saying do not swallow, while In US, paraphrasing, it will read, *poison, do not swallow, if swallowed contact your poison control centre.* Even the UK's British dental foundation cites on its FAQ's; *Children should be supervised up to the age of 7, and you should make sure that they spit out the toothpaste and do not swallow any if possible.*

Sure, Fluoride will kill pathogens and bugs that cause gum disease, it ought to, and it is after all a germicide and does kill rats! Worst still, once fluoride gets into the system it becomes almost impossible to rid the body of it completely. The EFSA quotes *"Absorbed fluoride is partly retained in bone and partly excreted, predominantly via the kidney. In infants retention in bone can be as high as 90% of the absorbed amount, whereas in adults retention is 50% or less".*[30]

The International Chemical Safety Cards reports the following[31]

Inhalation	Cough. Sore throat.
Ingestion	Redness.
Eyes	Redness. Pain.
Skin	Abdominal pain. Burning sensation. Convulsions. Drowsiness. Cough. Diarrhoea. Sore throat. Vomiting. Unconsciousness.

Below we can identify toothpastes containing the various degrees of fluoride added

Brand	PPM of Sodium Fluoride
Aquafresh	1450ppm
Crest Complete	1450ppm
Colgate Regular	1450ppm
Colgate Triple Action	1450ppm
Colgate Duraphat (prescription only)	2800ppm
Colgate Duraphat (prescription only)	5000ppm
Macleans Fresh Mint	1450ppm
Signal Family Protection	1450ppm

As you can see we are almost at the safety upper limit of 1500 ppm and the story does not end there. We now have to consider Hexafluorosilicic acid the fluoride added to water and now fluoride that is added to food supplies.

Hexafluorosilicic Acid

This is added to tap water to "cleanse" and make the water safe to drink. It is a fluorine and therefore a toxic chemical. As you might expect it is an inorganic compound and is a by-product of hydrogen fluoride and phosphate fertilizers, it is mainly used in the production of Aluminium! The International Chemical Safety Cards reports the following.

Inhalation	Burning sensation. Cough. Laboured breathing. Shortness of breath. Symptoms may be delayed.
Ingestion	Burning sensation. Abdominal cramps. Vomiting. Shock or collapse.
Eyes	Redness. Pain. Severe deep burns.
Skin	Redness. Pain. Skin burns.

Despite increasing evidence against proving that fluoride does not prevent dental carries or prevent disease, various governments have chosen to and therefore endorsed different maximum levels of fluoride to be added to the water supply and thus we can expect typically 1ppm. However Austria, Belgium, Denmark, Finland, Iceland, Holland, Italy and Sweden have no fluoride program for their water supply while Germany, Switzerland (Zurich) and France do add fluoride salt to the supply.

So the question's we must ask ourselves is: Why is there a poison warning on the product? Why does the government allow poison to be legal? Who says that fluoride prevents dental carries and gum disease? Where does the buck stop? The last question is easy to answer. For example, Andy Burnham former UK health secretary had a policy in place to fluoridate the UK's drinking water supply, the problem was that he forgot to inform the Parliamentary Register of Members' Interests that he was in fact the vice president of British Fluoridation Society, he hastily resigned his post at BFS.

The debate in Australia, Canada, USA and the UK is on-going as the fluoride companies push for further fluoridation in states, districts and region that have not already been poisoned!

What are the dangers of Fluoride use?

Bizarre as it may seem, Fluoride was at one time regarded as an essential nutrient![32]

Now it seems that is no longer the case, a blow to the fluoride industry, but their legacy and big bucks have bought legislation allowing more and more food, drink and medicine to contain toxic fluoride, all this in spite of damning independent research. Perhaps more research papers are available on this subject more than any other.

Research papers on Fluoride can be found at:

www.fluoridealert.com

http://www.ncbi.nlm.nih.gov

(Type in key words)

www.who.int (type in key words)

http://www.who.int/foodsafety/foodborne

_disease/chemicals.pdf
http://www.nap.edu/openbook.php?record_id=2204&page=1
http://scholar.google.com (type in key words)

Some articles from the press and leading fluoride awareness websites:

- Fluoride water 'causes cancer' Boys at risk from bone tumours, shock research reveals.[33] (The Guardian)
- Health Canada. Fluoride in Drinking Water.[34] (Fluoride alert)
- Chemicals used in the UK for fluoridation of public water supplies.[35] (BFS website)
- Scientific Facts on the Biological Effects of Fluorides.[36] (What the problem is)
- Top fluoride expert apologizes for pushing poison.[37] (Healthy communications)
- Sodium fluoride– toxicological overview.[38] (Environmental protection agency)

So you wash your teeth twice a day with Fluoridated toothpaste, you will absorb this into the system without swallowing it. You drink your tap or bottled water containing fluoride. Is that where it ends? No chance. If you are drinking soda and other commercially made drinks produced in an area where the water is fluoridated then you naturally increasing your intake, likewise with commercially prepared foods. Is that where fluoride intake ends?

Are you on medication? Depending where you live in the world you are probably ingestion more fluoride, especially if you are taking a certain strength Aspirin. Remember that fluoridated toothpaste instructs you **not to swallow!**

In many parts of the world you can find fluoride added to these consumer goods:

Medications	Food & Nutrition
Anesthetics (general)	Children's milk

Anti-fungal Antibiotics	Foods sprayed With pesticides
Antacids Antihistamines	Food supplements (sodium monofluorophosphate)
Arthritis (rheumatoid)	Petfood
Antibiotics (Fluoroquinolones)	Processed foods
http://www.slweb.org/ftrcfluorinatedpharm.html	Salt
	Water

Other products containing fluoride:

Ammonium Bi Fluoride

Bactericide in sugar industry

Ammonium Silico Fluoride

Etching glass

Chromium Fluoride

Dyeing and printing wool, paint primer for steel.

Sodium Fluoride

A steel degassing agent, disinfecting fermentation apparatus in breweries and distilleries, foundry fluxes, frosting glass, heat-treating salt compositions, preserving wood, manufacture of coated paper.

Sodium Bi Fluoride

A "sour" in laundering, electroplating

Sodium Fluoborate

Flux for Aluminium, flame retardant for Cotton and Rayon.

Potassium Fluoride

Catalyst for molds for dentures, component in Grinding Wheel, organic synthesis for introduction of Fluorine

Sodium Lauryl Sulphate

As you might expect by now, Sodium Lauryl Sulphate or SLS comes in around 150 guises the most popular being Sodium Laureth Sulfate, Sodium monododecyl sulphate, Sodium myreth sulphate & Sodium pareth sulphate & Amonium lauryl sulphate.

It is found in healthcare products such as soaps, shampoos and bubble baths, industrially it is used as engine degreasers and used in commercial car washes. It is highly corrosive and readily attacks greasy surfaces and therefore it is used as a degreasing agent in the cleaning of commercial floors.

Clinical use for SLS is used almost universally as a prime skin irritant. Laboratories use it on test animals and humans to test healing agents used in healthcare creams to see how effective an agent it is on the test subject.

If you are on medication look out. Many drugs that are poorly soluble in water will contain SLS to help the medicine go down!

Exposure to SLS can lead to Breathlessness, coughing, diarrhoea, headaches, irritating to the respiratory tract, nausea, redness and pain on the eyes and skin, sore throat & Vomiting. In extreme cases it can cause blindness. Science has proven that this compound damages protein in the eye tissues.

Extreme caution should be taken if you choose to apply SLS to your body. It can penetrate the brain and liver and remains there long term whilst degenerating cell brain membranes. Because it is a mutagen it can change genetic information in your cells and as a consequence harm your immune system.

SLS can cause hair loss by attacking the follicles and removes the body's natural oil from the skin. Since it is so corrosive it can peel away the top layer of skin on the scalp, a contributory factor to dandruff.

A study from The American journal of toxicology summarized its findings on long term use of SLS declaring that *"continued use of SLS and ALS appear not to be safe. Concentrations should not exceed 1-2% but most shampoos and conditioners, gels and creams contain between 10 - 20%."*[39]

In a later study the AJT reported that short term use (discontinuous) appeared to present less potential hazard on condition that it is thoroughly rinsed from the surface. As a footnote the study pointed out that carcinogenic nitrate can be formed in the manufacturing of SLS or by its reaction with other nitrogen bearing ingredients.[41]

The golden rule is to avoid as many

products as you can that contain the lauryl or laureth sulphate products. Like Fluoride it will not be easy, but make a start, the first an obvious place to begin would be to read the label, speak to a naturopath or better still do just a little research of your own and get proactive!

Below is a table showing some widely available and dangerous chemicals used in our everyday health products. These are but a few.

Chemical	Comp;osition	Use	Reaction
Acetaldehyde – a chemical intermediate for the production of acetic acid, esters and other chemicals.	A gas or colourless liquid, extremely flammable.	Nail polish remover.	Coughing, known carcinogen, Diarrhoea. Dizziness. Nausea, redness, Vomiting.
Alpha Hydroxy Acid – Used as a chemical peel.	A colourless hygroscopic crystals.	Anti-aging products.	Abdominal pain, burning sensation. Collapse, Cough, shortness of breath. sore throat. Destroys the cells (skin)

			making it more susceptible to even more damage.
Acetone – (Dimethylketone,2-Propanone, Beta-Ketopropane).	A colourless, volatile liquid with a pungent odour. Extremely flammable.	Nail polish remover.	Confusion, eye, headaches, lung, nose, throat irritant, long-term exposure includes increased birth defects, kidney, liver and nerve damage.
Bentonite – used as bonding, plasticizing, and suspending agent.	Soft clay that expands.	Shines the skin by bringing water to the surface.	Combustible, prevents normal oxygen respiration.
Bisphenol A - found in plastics and water bottles.	White crystals.	Helps shape and keep plastic together.	Considerable and various problems with constant use.
Dioxin – Used in agent orange.	Liquid.	Used in plastics – sewage sludge – Do not eat fish found near coast line.	Responsible for all types of diseases.
Ethylene glycol - Acrylic paints, antifreeze, brake fluid, tile grout,	In its purist form it is an odourless, colourless,	Used as a firming moisturizer and is used in	Backache, can cause drowsiness, & slurred speech

primer, sealant paste, floor polish.	syrupy, sweet-Tasting liquid.	some Soothing lotions.	& throat irritation, headache, kidney problems, oedema.
Gelatine – Made from the connective and skin tissue of pigs.	Various.	Used in certain foods as a gelling agent. In medicine it is used to manufacture capsules.	CJD (very low risk), Allergic reactions, bloating, belching, heartburn, and unpleasant taste.
Glycerine - A plasticiser and a solvent.	Syrupy liquid.	Skin moisturizer.	Takes water from the lower layers to the top as a consequence it ends up drying the skin.
Mineral Oil – Derives from pertoleum.	Oil.	Blush, baby oil, creams, foundation & lotions.	Blocks the pores and prevents toxins from leaving. Prevents Vitamin A absorption.
Parabens (synthetic).	Liquid.	Preservative found in cosmetics, medicine (approx. 400), some	Linked with breast tumours & cancer.

		food and drugs and toiletries.	
Phthalates - flooring, plastic, vinyl, wallpaper.	Materials that are derived from the organic chemical phthalic acid.	Deodorant, hair spray & gels, perfume, lotions & nail polish.	Kidneys, liver, lungs, and reproductive systems damage.
Polypropylene - used in carp parts, moulding, medical instruments, plastics and synthetic materials	A gas, resin. a simple chemical component of petroleum.	Cosmetics and soap and food containers.	Can be carcinogenic.
Propylene Glycol - brake and hydraulic fluid and industrial antifreeze	A colourless, volatile, flammable liquid produced by fermentation of yeast and carbohydrates.	Retains moisture in the skin by preventing the escape of moisture or water.	A strong skin irritant and can cause liver abnormalities and kidney damage.

So by now I hope that I have been able to illustrate clearly the bigger picture developing. It is about the money, it is always about the money and while the big corporations do not want you dead or sick in a way that can lead to your death or illness back to them, they certainly put their big bucks to use through lobbying, having laws passed in their favour making sure that their product is placed on the shelves in one form or another. Of course they know full well that there are safer and cheaper products that work effectively without their toxic poisons and we shall take a look at these in the chapter Non toxic alternatives.

NON TOXIC ALTERNATIVES

Not poisonous, harmful, or otherwise destructive to an organism.

Now we have discovered some problematic toxins in our everyday healthcare and sanitation needs. So what are the alternatives? There are many, it requires only a change of mind-set and a readiness to throw out the old and bring in the new. It is that simple. Really!

Sweeteners

Presuming that you do not have blood sugar problems, there are numerous alternatives to Aspartame and white refined sugar.

If sugar is a must then unrefined brown raw cane sugar is one alternative. It is natural and produced as nature intended containing approximately 50 calories per tablespoon. Check the label, it should read only as; raw cane sugar. One tablespoon of brown sugar is equal to that of around 50 calories while one tablespoon unrefined white sugar is that of around forty eight calories.

The table below shows some healthier alternative sweeteners that processed sweeteners including white sugar do not offer.

Blackstrap molasses ½ tablespoon = 25 calories	Strong flavour so you can reduce your sugar intake, contains calcium, magnesium, potassium, and iron, can help fight bad Cholesterol.
Manuka honey 1 tablespoon = 60 calories	Used in many countries for healing burns. Contains many anti-microbial and anti-bacterial properties. Helps heal and prevent throat disease. Helps gastrointestinal system, Heartburn, diarrhoea.
Maple syrup 1 tablespoon = 100 calories	Contains fewer calories than sugar, has high concentrations of Manganese and Zinc.
Stevia virtually no calories	Banned in some countries as a standalone sweetener. Helps regulate blood sugar, can aid in weight loss and weight management as it contains no calories, reduces sweet cravings.
Xylitol 1 tablespoon = 30 calories	Naturally found in the human body, fruits and plants. Mirrors sugar properties, it helps fight bacteria

	thus prevents cavities, helps weight loss, contributes to increased bone density.

Chlorine

Chlorine, now widely used is still avoidable. Unfortunately it comes down to budget. But even on a squeezed budget we can still address the problem. The first place to start would be to buy a chlorine filter which knocks out about 90% of the chlorine. They cost around £50.00 or $75.00s and remain effective for years. Especially in the shower as with heat, the toxic gases from chlorine are released. But if a filter is out of the question then you should not shower with the water steaming hot and have the bathroom well ventilated.

Drinking chlorine free water is less problematic as there are many portable water filter systems available such as Brita. Alternatively you can buy mineral water just make sure it contains no Aluminium or fluoride. Finally you can boil tap water vigorously, let it cool and bottle it in a glass bottle and refrigerate it. You might want to consider also taking a complement of minerals also.

Fluoride

As with chlorine, there are filters you can buy to remove fluoride from the water, they are considerably more expensive but if affordable then they are well worth the money. A reverse osmosis machine will also do the job. Some believe that since the osmosis process removes everything from the water, you are therefore drinking dead water with no mineral content. Once again this can be addressed by taking a complement of minerals with your exceptionally pure drinking water!

Fluoride free toothpastes are now becoming more common place. The added benefit of buying these products are that they will almost certainly be free of SLS, parabens, phthalates and artificial sweeteners, petrochemicals and colourants. Some are even being sold in the regular superstores. Obviously look online for your nearest supplier or buy online, your local independent health shop will almost certainly have them.

Consider only after seeking professional advice, clean your teeth by making 3% hydrogen peroxide from 35% food grade, mix this with Bicarbonate of soda to make a paste brush and then rinse your mouth with a homemade spearmint mouthwash. Simply buy some organic spearmint, steep it in very warm water for 30 minutes, bottle and keep out of sunlight. Perfect!

Sodium Lauryl Sulphate

Soaps and shampoos are now readily available without SLS and other chemicals. The golden rule is more equals less. The less ingredients in the soap and shampoo the better off you will be. Soaps traditionally add various perfumes, this is to disguise the smell of the chemicals used in the manufacturing process. You should consider soap derived from vegetable oil such as coconut oil or olive oil and not from animal fats and WITHOUT perfumes or scents. Even some organic soap will contain SLS as this is what is used to make the lather, you have to make a judgement call, and only you can make this call otherwise the alternative to washing with soap without absolutely no chemicals whatsoever is to manufacture your own.

Glycerine

The alternative skin moisturizers to Glycerine are many fold. It may not be exotic sounding but keeping your body fully hydrated with good quality water will naturally keep your skin hydrated, and you can supplement this by applying ozone oil, which will release oxygen into the applied area in a time fashioned manor. Rub on before you go to bed it will work its miracle of oxygenating cells without you even noticing. Shea butter, another excellent product with the added bonus of getting supplements of vitamin A & E. Aloe Vera, one of those wonderfully natural products that serve many uses. As a moisturizer it also soothes and softens. Coconut oil is one of the oldest and trusted skin moisturizers available, it is especially good for dry skin as it is absorbed into the skin speedily.

Parabens

A preservative found in cosmetics, medicine (approx. 400) and some food and drugs and toiletries. There is no short cut in buying products without this highly toxic chemical. You simply have to buy products derived from organic, oil or mineral based elements. Reading the label is essential and more importantly understanding what is not on the label. Another golden rule to follow is if you cannot eat it then do not put it on your skin! If parabens are in drugs you are taking, then inform your healthcare professional and ask him to find an alternative, paraben free.

Bisphenol A, Dioxin and Phalites

All found in plastic and from a consumer choice point of you there is absolutely no need for us to buy or accept any, but any product containing disease manufacturing chemicals.

Another golden rule. If man made it, don't touch it!

And so this rationale can be extended in consideration of hair sprays, nail varnish remover, perfumes, after shaves and deodorants. In most cases just a little thought is required before making your purchase. There are no longer any excuses; you can have all the cosmetics that you have been using up to now but without delivering poisons to your body. Visit natural health and mind body exhibitions and read specialist magazines to find what you are looking for. If free time is the problem, do an online search, it will not take very long, time yourself.

Confucious said. *"A journey of a thousand miles begins with a single step"*, take that single step today. Go for it! Today, throw away just one toxic item, one poison from the toxic overload your body been encumbered with up to now. Tomorrow or the day after, dispose of another and shortly after, another, enjoy yourself, why not perform an out with the old and in with the new ritual with a promise to yourself choosing a simple but effective affirmation.

EMOTIONAL AND PHYSICAL STRESS

A physical, mental, or emotional response to events that causes bodily or mental tension.

Perhaps one of the most underestimated aspects of our health is the role of the mind. We do know that an emotion can bring on a physical reaction and in fact some forward thinking scientists are now convinced that disease starts from outside our body as a cause of our thoughts. It is worth noting this aspect and bearing it in mind for future reference, but in this book we will address issues that are more certain.

The body has effectively two systems, the sympathetic otherwise known as the fight or flight system and the parasympathetic system, the rest and digest, the actual words or phrases are not important only their action.

Steeped in our primitive and biological history these two systems are designed for our survival.

The sympathetic system works by

deciding to stay and fight off an offender. A surge of adrenaline and other chemicals such as noradrenaline and cortisol are released into our bloodstream and are rushed to our arms and hands to give us the strength and energy for the oncoming fight. Our vision sharpens, our purpose becomes more resolved, impulses accelerate, our awareness becomes acuter and our ability to suffer pain increases.

On the other hand should we choose to run or take flight, then we are blessed with the same surge of adrenaline to the legs to give us the speed required to take flight from our attackers to maintain survival.

Staying in this mode is somewhat easy as our western lifestyles of worrying about maintaining our job, stress at work, financial problems, arguments, discord and undue worrying over our children's wellbeing are all modern day symptoms of the sympathetic mode. This is one place that you do not want to be for very long periods!

Long term use of this mode is damaging as:

- Blood is drawn away from our digestive tract and this is one reason why we have indigestion when we eat during or after an argument.
- We breathe shallow from the upper chest thus insufficient oxygen is carried to the lungs resulting in breathlessness, headache, a feeling of euphoria and nausea otherwise known as hypoxia.
- It can lead to high blood pressure.
- Attention span and our ability concentrate or focus on anything other than the "stressor" for a period of time is greatly reduced.
- In prolonged periods it can lead to heart disease and cancer.

(see table at the end of this chapter for other conditions)

A typical physical symptom of flight or flight would be after having had a big bust up with your loved one, often you can experience a knot in the stomach, it is very real, a stress hormone Cortisol has shut off the stomach and this is the knot sensation you feel.

Those women who are unable to conceive yet desperately want to conceive live in the fight or flight mode in the form of phantom pregnancy, they have managed to trick the brain into believing they are pregnant and experience the full complement of responses. Morning sickness, expanding stomach, periods stop, and the breasts enlarge. Unfortunately after nine months nothing happens except a lot of air is expelled resulting in immense disappointment together with psychological disorders albeit temporarily.

As a side note it is worth taking a moment to note the power of the mind. Many of whom have lost a limb experience Phantom Limb Syndrome while an exceptional Doctor by the name of Leonard Coldwell, now retired, as reported by two European independent studies has cured well over 35,000 people from cancer, a 92% success rate using no drugs, lotions or potions, but simply used methods that he devised to get you out of fight of flight, rid you of stress to allow the body's natural healing responses to perform.

Short term use of fight or flight can have some positive attributions. Sportsman use it, it gives them the edge, that fighting spirit and we often call on fight or flight to help us perform a task more readily and speedily and quite often musicians while composing get those rush of idea's and cannot stop to eat or answer the phone while their hand or computer keyboard tries impossibly to keep pace with fast thoughts of inspirational music flowing through their mind.

For good health we need to spend most of our time in the parasympathetic mode. This it seems we are finding more and more difficult to do, however we need to address the problem and no better place to start is other than breathing.

To breathe correctly just look at a babe in arms, they have not yet experienced stress or trauma, perhaps except for their experience of birth and even then they have not yet learned the craft of hanging on to the stress or fear of that experience. The babe you will recognize breathes in from the nose sending a supply of oxygen more readily to the brain and lungs whilst pushing out the abdomen. A deep intake of breath lasting around five seconds is relaxed and natural with no thought attached to the action followed by an equal measure of out breath through the mouth while bringing the stomach in. Now, watch an adult breath, most will breathe in with their mouth, (partially due to the bodily response of the disgusting odours of city life) while bringing in their stomach and again breathe out with their mouth simultaneously pushing out he stomach.

So we need to relearn how to breathe and there is a simple technique that you can call on to do this, whether sitting on a bus or lying in bed or while you are giving a public address in front of hundreds of people. Simply put one hand over your stomach, and instantly you will breathe while pushing out your stomach and you will start to breathe a little deeper, so simple. But this is a short turn problem to the solution and often we need assistance and sitting down on your own for ten minutes in a quiet room without TV or radio, in silence just concentrate on the correct breathing technique as do babes, think of some positive and pleasant thoughts to keep you in the parasympathetic mode. Well, I have just described to you the beginnings of meditation, (to know thyself) of course the person serious about meditation will need to attend classes and learn the various techniques from which they will find a suitable method for their individual needs. But in many cases learning the art of slowing down or switching off from the stress coupled with their own form of meditation is sufficient. It is not always that easy to simply switch off or have the patience to meditate or even just keep quiet for a few moments, you may be angry, frustrated or even have developed a low attention span in which case seeking professional help may be the answer, if meditation is something you feel is not suitable for you in your present state of mind then you might like to try Emotional Freedom Technique. A simple technique of tapping on certain points on the body from a pre written script ready for you to fill in the blanks for your individual needs and it is very, very effective. Many soldiers coming back from the various battlefields around the world have experienced Post Traumatic Stress Disorder (PTSD) and through EFT have conquered their anxieties. There are trained professionals in EFT but why not go the full nine yards and speak with Olivia Roberts at Resolution Magic who has taken the EFT technique and brought it to a different dimension. You can download free simple techniques of EFT to use yourself, more on this subject can be found in the last chapter of the book where we discuss the various therapies and protocols.

The process of relaxation can be aided further by ultimately abandoning the TV and radio while you are eating. Be more selective about the types of broadcasts you listen to and what journals you read. Are they all negative? Are the topics about war and violence, celebrity relationship bust ups? Or maybe just idol gossip columns. Choose something creative or humorous, we do know that laughing releases healing chemicals in the body called endorphins, these are the body's natural Pain killers that will aid any ailment that you are trying to recover from. Likewise watching the news or depressing soaps will have the adverse effect as this puts us directly back in the fight or flight mode, inhibits breathing and creates a negative ambiance in our life as daily doses become our living reality, just listen to how often we talk about "the news"! Interestingly the word endorphin comes from the Greek words endogenous + morphine endo (from within) + morphine (pain killer). Imagine that, we have our own supply of non-addictive Morphine in ready supply waiting to be released from our brain on command!

Other activities that can help us in healing are:

- Take walks in the countryside or in the park, just being outside in the sunshine (whenever possible) and around nature has a massive impact on our wellbeing. Walk barefoot in nature and heal Arthritis into the bargain. The earth's magnetic field reduces inflammation, fact!
- A recent article from the journal of Dr. William Douglas MD showed children with ADHD need no drugs, they simply need to stop eating junk food full of chemicals that unbalance the body's natural rhythm and to be in nature, walking, playing, and keeping the body moving.
- And this is something we can once again learn from babies, to be joyous, cheerful and playful as these simple and natural techniques in time will lighten your load, change your perspective or current viewpoint of life and consequently change your attitude towards problems. Talk about relieving

stress and it did not cost a dime!

- Enjoy a weekly massage to relieve yourself from those physical aches and pains that you encumbered at work.
- Join an association that shares your interests and interact with other people, get involved, get active! Take the step now! What are you waiting for!
- Take the time to resolve issues with friends and family, but truly resolve issues not just the mere words, really feel it and watch your physical symptoms disappear. This is where EFT can really help you to resolve unresolvable issues.

Like attracts like and as hard as it may seem, you really need to keep away from people who are negative, those that find fault in everything, the prophets of doom and gloom, some of them are at work but you simply cannot pack in your job as you have acquired many obligations on your journey of life that needs to be supported by finance, but by changing your mind-set and therefore your approach to how you deal with it, you can simply acknowledge the moans and groans without fuelling it with your own comments. Be aware of this and try it out next time and after you have resisted commenting, notice how you feel, it may be subtle but you will feel emotionally better and with practice this feeling of wellbeing gets stronger and stronger. Having said all this maybe your husband, wife, children or long term partner is contributing to the stress and consequently physical conditions and you just cannot walk out, neither should you, this is where you need to sit down, talk it through and find some common ground and maybe get some professional help.

The root of the problem though, lies within you! You cannot control what people do or say but you can control how you act or react to them. All of us need to face our demons to move forward physically, spiritually and emotionally. Can you look yourself in the eye in a mirror and confront yourself with a specific problem, without being angry with yourself or without turning away? Try it and see. Once you can do this you are the right place to start healing and enjoying good health.

Anger/Hate ➔ acidic body ➔ breeding ground for disease

Love ➔ PH neutral body ➔ healing & health

The link between emotional stress and physical symptoms are well established and documented. Appreciating we are all unique, the emotional state of mind may for example introduce the imbalance Arthritis to one individual yet may not do the same to another, it may in fact induce back pain The table overleaf indicates some typical mind / physical relationships.

AIDS	Inability to self-love, accept gender, low self-esteem, permanent sense of guilt, self-punishment (emotionally).
Anxiety	Breathing problems, light-headedness, Nausea, palpitations, sweating, shaking, stomach knots, swallowing (difficulty).
Arthritis	Depression, stress.
Asthma	Anger, birth trauma, crying, laughing, panic, suffocating relationships (including unresolved parent issues).
Back pain	Depression, fear, stress, trauma.
Bladder	Anxiety, dread, fear, inadequacy, panic.
Cancer	Stress, feeling of helplessness, repressing emotions.
Eczema	Anger, sadness, stress, suppressed emotions, trauma,
Heart disease	Anger, frustration, hate, excessive excitability &

	hysteria, irritation, low self-esteem, stress.
Kidney disease	Fear, inability to let go.
Lung disease	Anxiety, depression, grief, sadness.
Migraine	Anger, excitement, disappointment, mental disharmony, rage.

ELECTROMAGNETIC CHAOS

The invisible electromagnetic radiation from wireless technology and mains electricity.

A relatively new phenomenon that we are just beginning to understand and we simply cannot avoid it, so we have to deal with it. Cell phone towers and cell phones, Wifi signals, wireless modems, smart meters and even good old fashioned electricity has found to have presented problems and until recent years it was not recognized as a problem, but a few years down the line and after many studies we now know why there are higher Leukaemia rates in certain areas, brain tumours are on the increase, well why wouldn't there be, should we be surprised? After many years of sticking a wireless headset in your ear you are getting full on radiation going straight in your ear drum!

Do you find that when you are in a particular person's home that you do not feel well, you feel sick, nauseous, headaches, problems focusing and you want to leave and when you do the problems disappear? You have just experienced Sick House Syndrome and you may have been experiencing this in your own home but were unable to understand why you feel sick in your own home!

And there is no escape in the park either, if you can get online then you will be increasing your daily dose of radiation likewise the many passers-by who are sitting around you. Coffee shops and even the metro in some countries allow these wireless signals to penetrate.

The main problem lies once again with flawed research and so we have to consider the individual, how much time do you spend on a cell phone, this may-be somewhat minimal but if you live in an apartment with cell towers on the roof, then you may have a problem re-enforced if you leave your wireless router on in your home 24/7, worst still leaving it on in your bedroom while you sleep!

All this wonderful technology that we rely

on is here to stay but we simply cannot continue to use it in the way that we have been doing. Once again we need address the problems and take some simple precautions to in most cases resolve the issues, others may need more drastic measures such as moving home.

Cell Phones

Children are more at danger when using mobile phones as their skull is not fully developed; a five year olds skull is much thinner than an adult's skull so consequently through the ear drum they can absorb up to 50% more radiation than

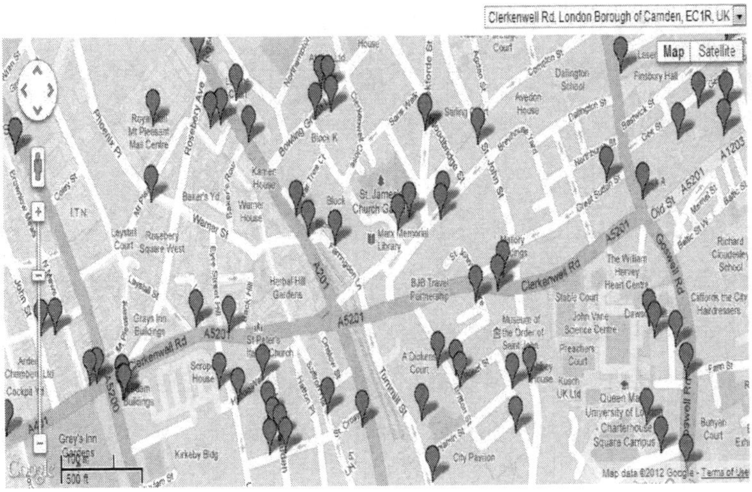

adults. This absorption rate decreases to about 30% as they get older (ten years) An Australian study in 2004 revealed that radiofrequency radiations (RFR) which included mobile phones remained uncertain about their safety and concluded that *"RFR from mobile phones can cause peripheral neurophysiological changes in some persons. The effects occur at exposure levels below the present safety levels for RFR."* [41]

The debate on safety of cell phones has undergone vigorous scrutiny. Nearly all independent studies indicate that cellular phone use under certain conditions, such as remaining on the phone for too long, remaining on the phone for prolonged periods when the signal bar is low and so on pose dangers ranging from neurological disorders to blood pressure problems and cancer. However nearly all the industry based studies or government reports state that there is no evidence to support cell phone use is hazardous for short term use and they are very cautious about risk analysis with long term use. Why is this?

Why are there such obvious contradictions? The answer is pretty obvious also. From 1990 – 2010 global cell subscriptions grew from 12.4 million to over 4.6 billion.[42] That is a lot of income, a lot of jobs and a lot of tax revenue being collected. With so much data readily available it is therefore more practical to address the issues in table below rather than site endless supporting studies. The risks shown are generally for excessive and continuous use and as I have continually mentioned in this book, we are all individual, we are all unique and these risk factors increase depending on your own set of circumstances.

Cell Phone Risks

Alzheimer's, MS & Parkinson's disease	Caused by proteins and toxins leaking into the brain.
Blindness	Breaks blood brain barrier, risk of blindness due to clotting.

Blood pressure	10-15mm Hg average increase in blood pressure. Could be dangerous if you already have high blood pressure.
Cancer	Increased risk of brain cancer and tumours on the side of the brain where you use the phone.
DNA damage	Can lead to the formation of tumours and cancer, cell suicide or take over the cell structure.
Headaches	Often starting immediately but also follows later in the day.
Heart disease	Radiation causes red blood cells to leak haemoglobin.
Mind	Changes the neurology of the brain.

Cell Phone Masts

Many people living near cell masts are experiencing problems, sometimes we can define this under Sick house syndrome. Power watch reported that the cancer rate, not cancer risk but

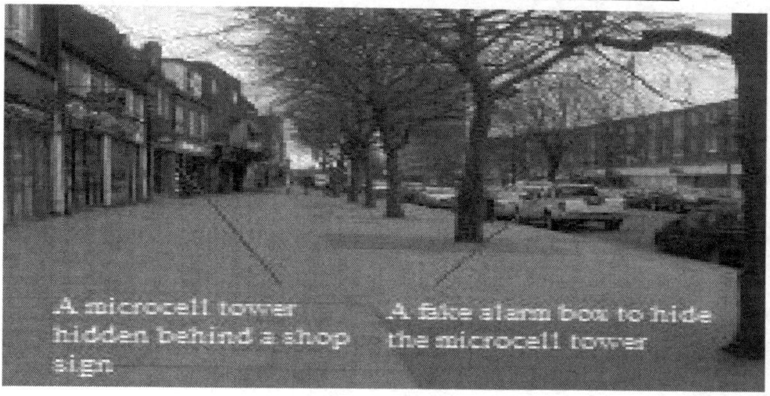
A microcell tower hidden behind a shop sign
A fake alarm box to hide the microcell tower

cancer rate increased just over four times for those living around 350 metres of a phone mast for between three to seven years, compared to the rate found overall in people living in the nearby town of Netanya, Israel. Women were worst off, the “risk” of cancer increased tenfold. There are so many of these masts on top of buildings, usually but not exclusively in a work environment that nobody notices them anymore, they are in fact hidden in plain sight! These cell masts emit around ten times the amount of radiation that of a microwave oven so naturally they present over and above the problems discussed with cell phone use, cell masts present their own unique problems. Children living near TV and FM towers (emitting similar radiation to cell towers) developed Leukaemia at three times the rate those living several miles away. Miscarriages are not uncommon and a notable sperm count drop in men has been reported.

The phone companies have figured out pretty quickly that we know these towers are not healthy and damn right dangerous and whilst on the one hand they seem to comply readily with the public outcries they are on the other

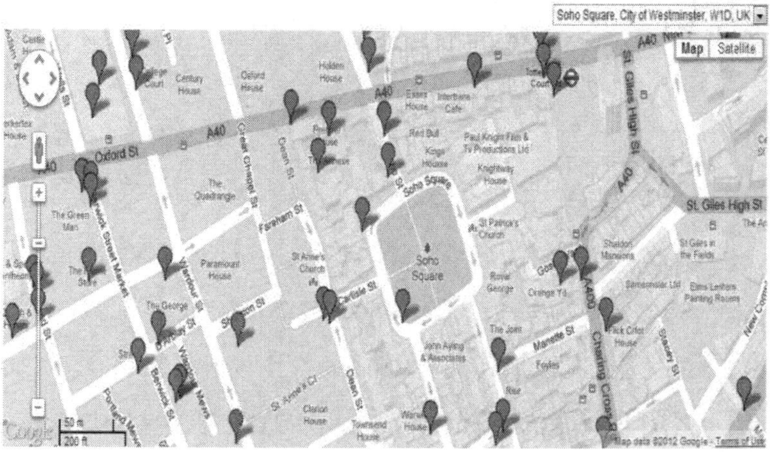

hand very sinisterly exploiting a loophole in the law by replacing these towers with micro base cells. These box shaped stations are mounted on lampposts and walls, they are even disguised as burglar alarms and hidden behind pub signs. The *loophole "De minimis non curat lex"*, or *"the law does not care about very small matters"* indicates perfectly local authority contempt for their tax paying citizens health as no planning permission is required for the masts if they are less than ten meters off the ground (only a 28 notice of installation required) thus making exposure to radiation from the masts even greater as they are much closer to us. On the last count in London's Soho, within a quarter of a sq mile there are 94 micro base cells and another 11 masts on top of buildings! Not an area of London you want to live, work or play in!

WIFI

Wireless another idea proving although very convenient, not such a good idea. Schools throughout the world are now choosing to remove wifi systems because the irrefutable independent studies condemning wifi as perilously dangerous. Absenteeism, headaches, attention deficit and low concentration span are high in schools with wifi throughout. As you would expect radiation exposure is top of the list, lungs, heart, eyes and thyroid glands all are susceptible to wifi radiation exposure.

So why do we continue to use wifi, again we must look at the industry and the wealth of tax revenue and jobs that are created. It is a sad fact but *"De minimis non curat lex"* is the appropriate phrase and our health concerns are low on the list.

The CTIA, the international association for wireless telecommunication industry explains perfectly the reasons for the growth in wireless communication. It will create over 200,000 jobs by 2015, $63 billion a year worldwide will be spent on wireless accessories. Businesses spent just under $2billion and is expected to top $5 billion by 2014, one of the fasted growing economic sectors growing of 16 % compared to other industries of just 3%. So these are the reasons for being radiated daily, it's all about the money and not health. Remember, *"De minimis non curat lex"* or "the law does not care about very small matters". I.e. OUR HEALTH!

Smart Meters

Another harmful source of energy, supposedly eco-friendly, but nothing could be further from the truth. I wrote an article on smart meters awhile ago and sums up perfectly what you can expect if you have one of these carcinogens installed in your home.

(Smart Meters – Cancer, personal surveillance & the de facto Eugenics program)

On the other hand there is an abundance of well documented studies that prove these "dirty, non-eco-friendly" meters of mass destruction are a clear and present danger to our health.

Lyon, France, May 31, 2011. The World Health Organization warns that Smart meter radiation is a Class 2B carcinogen. It is important to understand that this study was looking into the health effects of microwave radiation in general and not solely on smart meter radiation, however you mix it, the result is still the same.

Summarizing Daniel Hirsch senior lecturer on nuclear policy at UCSC (university college of Santa Cruz) said: *"The State legislator asked for an independent study as PG&E* (The Pacific Gas and Electric Company) *study concluded that there was nothing to worry about. Rightly, the state legislature wanted an independent study from a party that was uninterested in the outcome of the study".* He went on to say that what troubled him was that *"The CCST's* (California council on science and technology) *independent report was conducted by the Richard Tell the same person who compiled the initial report for*

PG&E. furthermore EPRI report (Electric Power Research Institute) *contained a table which CCST compared radiation doses from a smart meter, cell phone and a microwave oven".* Daniel Hirsch concluded by saying: *"The problem here is that they were comparing apples and oranges. They looked at whole body exposure from a smart meter and compared it to the dose to the ear from a cell phone instead of looking at the whole body dose from a cell phone and comparing it to the whole body dose of a smart meter. They also presumed 100% duty cycle for the smart meter and a 1% duty cycle for the cell phone where you are only using the cell phone for part of an hour a day on average. They did not correct for that, they did not look at the key motive exposure, 99% of the time the cell was not producing radiation but they assumed 100% of the time that the smart meter would, however when you correct for these two factors the smart meter turns out to be 100 times more key motive than the cell phone".*

The carcinogenic factor aside, these

meters are found to be partially responsible for Sick House Syndrome and there are endless testimonies on how headaches, Migraines and other neurological disorders miraculously disappear when smart meters are removed from the premises. Even MS suffers have found relief from their symptoms. A 2008 study by DR Magda Havas showed that the radiation waves can contribute to high blood sugar levels and that *"By closely following plasma glucose levels in four Type one and Type two diabetics, we find that they responded directly to the amount of dirty electricity in their environment"*.

Cardiac, Respiratory & Ophthalmologic problems are reported but since the smart meters are "approved" and adverse health effects take place over a long period of time, it is very difficult to make the power companies accountable for their equipment.

The power companies do not care about your health, their only agenda is to maximize profits. In 2010 PG&E in the last of cases linked to Erin Brockovich PG&E settled for $20 million. In October 2010 PG&E were hit by five several wrongful death lawsuits and most recently on September 01, a number of San Bruno residents sued PG&E over the deadly PG&E pipeline explosion.

And the list goes on and on and on!

Only when the last tree has died, the last river has been poisoned and the last fish has been caught will we realize that we cannot eat money – **Native Indian proverb**

Radiation

While we have been talking about radiation it should be noted that radiation can be leaked from radon gas, found naturally in the earth's crust, attributed as the largest contributor to background radiation doses that an individual can receive. In our modern hermetically sealed homes radon gas can accumulate in basements and lofts. It needs to be addressed as Radon is the foremost cause of lung cancer amongst non-smokers!

What is the safe and acceptable level of Radon gas in and around the home? The first part is easy to answer, no radon gas is the safest. But in reality many parts of whatever country you live will have higher, lower levels and no levels of Radon gas emissions. Each country has set its own safety standards and measurement terms. The USA sets a standard for indoor safety equal to that of what it believes is a safe outdoor upper limit of 0.4 pCi/L. (P = parts per trillion and CI = to curries and L stands for litre) In the Uk they have set the standard of 200 Bqm-3 (Becquerels per cubic meter)

Ironically the CI or curries in 0.4pc/l is named after Madame or Marie Currie, it was she who discovered that the harmful properties of radiation kill tumours and at low doses are used as an x ray to look inside the body. Ironic as knowing now what we know about the dangers of radiation, we have the Marie Currie cancer care centres all over UK to assist cancer patients who have gone through radio and chemotherapy.

To summarize, if your family has a history of cancer then you do increase your risks by excessive cell phone use, living near cell masts and an area that is even within the acceptable safety levels as laid down by law. But remember, your body only understands natural law, it does not care about legislative law on what are recommended safety levels on any issue and it will simply not be challenged on the matter, you cannot hoodwink or fool it, and your body knows exactly what is good and bad and will react accordingly, period!

PROTOCOLS, THERAPIES AND NATURAL MEDICINES

In other words, how to reverse disease naturally.

This part of the book is written in alphabetical order and it has been written purposely so since sharing with you the knowledge of protocols, therapies and treatments in any other order would almost certainly create a bias that could lead you to believe the treatments available at the start of the following section are more beneficial to you than those further along the directory and if you have followed the book thus far then it would be quite apparent that there is no one size fits all.

Other considerations have to be factored in. When selecting a natural treatment to resolve any imbalances then the financial implications have to be addressed as there is little money available from the public purse.

The following directory is quite comprehensive but not complete, there are many new discoveries coming online weekly and were either too late for print or while results look promising and report many success stories, more time, clinical results and testimonies are required.

Before you choose the protocol that you feel is best for you, you will no doubt make further research to verify efficacy, in doing so you will come across many websites that will ridicule, vilify and accuse natural remedies and protocols of quackery. Their research in order to justify the program may show some positive results on some natural products that have no real therapeutic value or have rewritten some text from a flawed study, but this is all a distraction. Typically these websites are often very slick corporate style designs with names that sound as though are part of an institution or a medical research facility.

Typically these spoof websites are named to give the impression that they are working for promoting natural medicine by giving themselves titles such as *The Natural Health Institute for Plant Medicine, The*

Amazon Medicine Research Lab, The National Institute for Health and Wellness, The Centre for Efficacy in Natural Medicine and so on.

One usual argument disclosed on these websites is that the natural product or protocol has not gone through the often flawed double blinded peer review process, the method largely accepted as the means to prove whether or not we benefit from reviewed test products. But what you are not told is that most of the natural remedies and protocols treat the whole body in order for the immune system and cleansing organs to be strong enough to reverse the disease of its own volition from the body's pool of cleansing and healing chemicals readily available.

Natural methods allow healing of the whole body using a variety of, for example, herbs or liquids synergistically such as MMS or DMSO. It would be impossible to produce biomarkers to track the progress of the medicine as there is so much happening at any one time. This of course is in opposition to drug medication trials which look at a single problem, say Arthritis, with a single drug. Under these conditions scientists can identify a biomarker and track the progress of the drug.

It is at this point you will need to remain resolute as it would be easy to fall back into the trap of believing that only drugs and surgery can cure.

The protocols therapies and natural medicines below are not designed to give in depth detail of the protocol itself but merely to give you an understanding of how they work. As always, caution and good knowledge of the protocol or advice should be taken before starting such a therapy and never stop taking any medication without speaking to your healthcare practitioner.

Alexander Technique

An educational discipline with therapeutic effects that teaches how to free oneself of self-imposed limitations unintentionally learned on the journey of life.

Strictly speaking AT is not a therapy but is exactly what is says it is, a technique. Perhaps one of the gentlest therapies available, generally there is no eureka moment for students as the therapy works over a period of time taught by a certified teacher.

Depending on what you expect to gain from the class will determine how many visits you will need. AT addresses posture enabling you to move in a more relaxed and comfortable way, the way nature intended. Classes do involve your participation but unlike yoga and other mediums there are no stretches or exercises involved and you do not take your clothes off.

Typically AT is known for assisting but not limited to people with:

- Backache
- Carpal Tunnel Syndrome
- Migraine and other cranial problems
- Repetitive Strain Injury
- Sitting down pains
- Stiff neck and shoulders
- Walking difficulties

Actors, athletes, dancers, singers, musicians all go to AT school to help them reach their full potential.

Lung cancer patients benefit from AT as the correct posture eases tension in the body and lungs allowing a better flow of oxygen. Fuller intake of oxygen reaches the brain which also improves cognitive abilities and can help you regain clarity of mind, essential for any healing process to take place, natural or drug related.

Pupils soon learn that their posture is linked to their emotional state of mind, consequently when you learn to walk, stand and sit as nature intended there becomes a shift in emotional and mental attitude.

Naturally, one benefit from this therapy is that you begin to feel good about your own body, thus the mind body link is realized.

It can be used as a standalone therapy or would work extremely well together with EFT (emotional freedom technique).

The Beck Protocol

A four part electro-medicine protocol that builds the immune system.

This electromagnetic medicine is used in four stages to disable or kill microbes, pathogens or bugs from multiplying in the body. Consequently it can be used for a host of ailments ranging from Aids, Arthritis, to Cancer and beyond. Once these microbes are neutralized, the immune system immediately becomes supercharged and kicks into action. The advantages of the beck protocol is that it can be used as a preventative treatment to maintain a good and strong healthy body, using the Beck protocol for a period of time (depending on your condition already) should leave you to get through the winter months without a cold or flu, certainly if you still caught a bug you would rid it from your body very, very, quickly. As with all natural therapy's, The Beck protocol reverses pretty much all bodily imbalances. HIV sufferers for whom this protocol was initially designed for have reported their viral loads decreasing and CD count up, there are many forums available where you can check out what users of this protocol are saying.

On the downside, for serious conditions such as Aids or cancer , you should not use this protocol once you start on prescription drugs or have started chemo or radiotherapy as a conflict can occur. Bob Beck wrote, *"First, for several days prior to starting this program, you must avoid ingesting anything containing medicinal herbs, foreign or domestic, or potentially toxic medication, nicotine, alcohol, recreational drugs, laxatives, tonics, garlic and certain potentially toxic vitamins, because blood electrification will cause electroporation, ..., which is lethal".*

You should not use or be on this protocol the same day as taking:

- Alcohol
- Blood thinners
- Coffee
- Enzymes
- Garlic
- Herbs

- OTC's
- Pain killers
- Supplements

Or when:

- Pregnant
- Using pacemakers
- Taking recreational drugs
- Smoking
- On supplements

This is a time consuming protocol and for serious conditions it takes about two to three months to really kick in, but if time is on your side then please note that this protocol is one of the most powerful natural non-invasive therapies available.

There may be some side effects if you go to fast to quick, nausea, detox rash also known as The Herxheimer reaction. This is a good reaction, it shows that the protocol is working.

This protocol offers nothing in the way of nutrition or nutrition based diets for specific conditions which essential in life threatening conditions such as AIDS or cancer and does not address the problems of nutritional deficiencies in Arthritis patients who continually eat processed foods. These people are just making the process harder and longer to be effective. If you keep doing what you are doing, you will keep getting what you get!

Ozonated Water

Drinking ozonated water is the perfect way to get oxygen into the body, anaerobes, pathogens and bugs cannot live in an oxygen rich environment, your blood and fluids get cleaned allowing easier transportation of nutrients and minerals and better communication between cells. Drinking ozonated water alone will not get rid of cancer or Aids alone but will also help keep infection down and slow the spreading of the disease to allow other parts of the protocol to do their job. (See ozone treatment for life threatening diseases).

Magnetic Pulser

The magnetic pulser is designed to search out and destroy microbes hidden in between tissues, the lymph system, root canals, the stomach area or those places you may find between a rock and a hard place, in other words MP is designed to destroy microbes not floating around in the blood stream.

You should use this until the machine has completed its factory set cycle. Use the MP before using the silver pulser as some of the microbes may disengage themselves from their hiding place and float around in the blood stream.

The Silver Pulser

The silver pulser or blood electrifier will disable microbes floating around the blood stream and should be used approximately 20 minutes after the magnetic pulser, and you should build up the amount of time you spend with this apparatus starting with ten minutes, the time it takes the blood to make a complete cycle of the body, and going up to and not exceeding 40 minutes over a period of weeks that you feel comfortable with, then you should slowly reduce your time period and do not drop from 40 minutes to 10 minutes in one day! Using this apparatus along with the ozonated water will restore your blood to the natural cherry red colour it ought to be.

Colloidal Silver

An antimicrobial nutrient it is also known as nature's antibiotic, (see colloidal silver for a more in-depth look) given time and in sufficient quantities it can kill the microbes in cancer cells thus allowing the cell to restore itself to a normal healthy cell. While it is a good idea to have small quantities of silver throughout the day (your vendor will be able to instruct you on this) it is essential to **stop drinking the silver 2 hours** before using the MP and SP and around 15 to 20 minutes after use. It is not dangerous only you will be using up its valuable resource when it could be used more effectively elsewhere. As a further precaution allow a short time to pass between drinking silver and ozonated water.

That concludes the four part Beck protocol.

Cymatics

Based on the theory that human cells, organs, and tissues have each a natural resonant frequency which changes when that part of the body is diseased.

One of many bio resonance therapies, naturally this protocol is unsupported by the traditional scientific thinking; nonetheless the use of Cymatics has a proven track record and in the hands of an experienced practitioner healing takes place. The principle of Cymatic therapy is that every healthy cell, organ and tissue has its own unique vibration and when that part of the body becomes diseased, the vibration changes. Cymatherapy provides precise combinations of frequencies that "shift" the imbalanced part of the body (rather than through the auditory canal) that are associated with healthy tissue and organ systems to that of its natural frequency and resonance. Therefore it does require the skill and experience of a trained practitioner.

Since this therapy works at cellular level where all disease takes place, as you would expect, it is capable of healing all body imbalances.

DMSO

Dimethyl Sulfoxide - A solvent with strong evidence of a wide variety of properties.

Regarded as the silver bullet of medicine in the 60's, DMSO became foul to the powers to be and its legal use by clinicians and physicians is greatly restricted. However as a private individual you are pretty much free to use it how you wish. Caution and knowledge is the rule!

DMSO has a variety of healing qualities. Top athletes are administered it by their teams physician to heal up sprains and bruises quicker than normal although he will never admit to it. It's anti-inflammatory properties can reduce swelling very quickly. Once applied topically it will absorb immediately into the skin, for this reason it is used as a carrier for other drugs. Those who are prescribed penicillin can ask the Doctor to inject some penicillin into a small amount DMSO, apply to the skin and The DMSO will bring the penicillin into the body with it without the need of inserting the needle into the body.

DMSO also helps medication cross the blood brain barrier, excellent if you are taking medication for brain conditions.

DMSO has also helped prevent paraplegia if administered quickly.

For topical applications 90% seems to work best, if you have fair skin or sensitive skin then you should use 70%, however studies have shown that the efficacy of 99.9% DMSO diminishes its healing capabilities on the body.

DMSO can also be applied intravenously and there are specialist Doctors, depending on what part of the world you live who are licensed to do so for certain conditions only.

DMT or DMSO Potentiation Therapy is used to allow chemo to target only cancerous cells, it's not a perfect solution but it does reduce the damage chemo creates more than significantly, as consequence far less chemo treatments would be required and notably less damage to the body.

DMSO can be used as a standalone treatment or adjunct to any other treatment or therapy, it really is the silver bullet of medicine.

There is perhaps one downside to this product, if you were to apply topically a small amount of DMSO on your foot, with in about 30 seconds you will have a garlic type taste in your mouth which may prove a problem in the work environment.

It is essential you know more about DMSO if only to have in the home as an antibacterial product. Please visit Dr. Stanley Jacob at www.dmso.org

EFT – Emotional Freedom Technique

A psychological / acupressure technique.

Along with The Alexander Technique and chi quong, EFT or Emotional Freedom Technique is one of the gentlest techniques/ therapies available. Based on the Chinese meridian energy system, emotional freedom relieves physical pain by gently tapping with the fingertips in certain areas of the body while making affirmations and as a consequence blocked energy is released and physical pain is relieved. The technique involves focusing on the issue be it physical or emotional and works well for people whose physical problems or their lack of ability to heal, are due to emotional problems. Often used but not exclusively by people with deep rooted physical pain and anger and returning soldiers with PTSD.

Since EFT works on unblocking emotional problems, it helps people with addictive behaviours, chronic conditions such as fatigue, fears, guilt, phobias, low self-esteem and stress.

There is much free information readily available that you can download on how to learn and practice EFT at home. A word of warning though, quite a few people give up or fail with home use as they become too impatient to learn the art of tapping or do not follow through the exact instructions or become undisciplined. Either way if you fall into this category and you are ready to admit it, then healing has begun and you should complete the process by visiting an EFT practitioner.

Gerson Therapy

A nutritional based therapy.

Arguably one of the most important breakthroughs in the fight against degenerative disorders with an extremely high rate of success, the Gerson therapy was originally developed for and cured many cases of advanced tuberculosis and naturally enough Dr. Max Gerson made further studies to treat infectious diseases, heart, chronic and other diseases including non-life threatening. The principle of this therapy is that of nutritional and cleansing of the whole body to allow a natural healing process to take place. The therapy includes drinking some 13 organic juices providing the body with an abundance of enzymes, vitamins and nutrients. The cleansing process includes up to three coffee enemas per day and drinking ozonated water plus three organic vegetarian meals per day. Fresh fruit and vegetables can be consumed all day along with certain supplements specific to your individual needs.

On the downside this therapy is probably the most expensive where a two week stay at their centre in Hungary would cost 5500 euro and double that in Tijuana, Mexico. It can be arduous and special juicing equipment is required should you choose to do this therapy at home. You cannot use this therapy if you have started chemo and you will probably not be accepted if you have a brain tumour due to swelling.

On the upside, independent testimonies have reported fabulous results especially with people who have stopped chemo and have been sent home to die. If cost is a factor you can apply this therapy via their home program and for the neediest they lend the expensive juicers and offer a home support team.

Before you say yea or nay to this therapy go to Google video and check the documentary *Dying to Have Known*.

Hemp Oil

Pressed from the seed of the hemp (cannabis) plant.

One of the most controversial healing products on the market. It is very difficult to obtain as depending on where you live in the world it is illegal. Often disregarded by some because of the association with "pot heads" and junkies. However this label is largely diminishing now and in California there are many legal dispensaries where you can buy hemp on prescription. Co-ops are also growing hemp for medicinal purposes.

But it is the hemp oil with THC (tetrahydrocannabinol) that is of interest here. Hemp oil is a powerful detoxifier and is a known cancer killer. The precise mechanism remains unclear but numerous studies prove this. Even so this natural product will also lower blood pressure and can rejuvenate vital organs such as the pancreas and accordingly many diabetics become "former diabetics" and insulin free. It is not an overnight process but can take up to around six weeks or perhaps longer for the healing to take place.

To begin with you should start with one dose three times per day building up to for serious conditions such as cancer, around 25 drops per day for around 5-6 weeks depending. Once again I have to stipulate there are no hard and fast rules; you have to reach your maximum dosage so that you feel comfortable. It is quite common for people to add some organic single and cold pressed extra virgin oil to make it more palatable and to aid in the dispensing of the hemp oil.

The oil has a relaxing effect and soon after administering the oil you will want to lie down and rest, some may say this is a side effect while others argue that rest is a very important part of the healing process.

It can play a supportive role with the use of chemo.

Other benefits include the prevention and relief of Arthritis, Asthma and Hypertension, Diabetes, Depression and Heart disease to name but a few.

Either way hemp seed should be added to salads as it is rich in EFA's (essential fatty acids) promote fluidity in the cells making it easier for nutrition to get in and junk to get out!

This product is quite difficult to obtain and those interested in using it should watch Rick Simpson's video Run from the cure at Phoenixtears.ca Here you will also learn how to make your own Hemp oil with THC, dosage information and a comprehensive look at how hemp oil works.

One last note on this oil, you can buy hemp oil almost universally in stores for salad dressings and alike but it will not contain any THC the active ingredient required for healing. Either way Hemp oil without THC is very beneficial to the overall function of the body.

Master Mineral Solution

A chemical oxidizer that has the ability to enter the body, kill pathogens that are causing diseases.

Ranked alongside hemp oil as one of the most controversial remedies, MMS formerly known as miracle mineral supplement was developed by Jim Humble, a prospector, to cure malaria. The principle of MMS is very simple and straightforward and can relieve symptom of certain imbalances within hours.

There are various protocols to be administered for various conditions but the principle Sodium Chlorite is activated with citric acid which becomes Chlorine Dioxide. Even though you see the name Chlorine it is absolutely not Chlorine, chlorine dioxide is something very different. The Chlorine Dioxide (NaC102) once swallowed creates Myeloperoxidase which the body's immune system uses to make Hypochlorous Acid. It is the Hypochlorous Acid that kills bugs, pathogens, viruses and diseased cells. Because our immune system is so clogged, we are unable to produce sufficient quantities HOCl and disease can manifest.

For serious conditions along with Dr. Simoncini's Bi carbonate of soda protocol this is the probably the most inexpensive protocols available for curing nearly all diseases, ALS still seems to be immune to this protocol although MMS does slow the degeneration process considerably. You can buy MMS legally although it would be sold as a water purifier only, alternatively you can make it yourself for pennies. There are also ministers of Jim Humbles' Genesis II church that will give you the MMS free although donations are welcome.

Only tiny drops of MMS are required, smaller doses more frequently have proven to be more beneficial than taken larger amounts.

As with most natural remedies you need to start slow and build up tolerance. If you feel nauseous, vomit or have diarrhoea then you know that the protocol is working, this is a good thing but it also means you have over done it.

MMS can be applied topically also by

spraying it on the desired part of the body. Applying DMSO will carry the MMS into the skin much quicker for faster results.

MMS can also be used for dental problems and some people use a special protocol for cleaning their teeth, a very powerful antibacterial.

On the downside, the taste to MMS is generally regarded as disgusting and this does put people off. But if you have a very tight budget then MMS is a protocol that should be looked at.

Much false information has been written about MMS, probably because it does work and costs the drug industry a lot of money as people who use MMS have no need for expensive medical procedures.

You should visit Jim Humbles websites[43] and sign up for his free regular newsletter[44] and most importantly visit the official MMS forum[45] where you can get all the free advice you need from MMS experts answering all your questions and concerns on MMS.

I would like to add here that please,

please do not be put off thinking that because this and other protocols like Dr. Simoncini's are so simple that they are not as good as they purport to be or that they are just quack treatments, that is what main stream medicine would like you to believe. Once you select a protocol, it is important to stick with it, be patient, changing midway will not achieve anything as you'll end up disappointed. Understand also that like drug medicine not all natural remedies work for any one individual, which is just the way it is!

Ozone Therapy

A variety of practices in which active oxygen is administered.

Tried, tested and used by medical doctors for many years throughout the world, yet remarkably the scientific community regard it as having no therapeutic value, some go on further to say that it is a toxic gas. However, there is so much data on the efficacy of ozone and its ability to rid the body of all imbalances that it is quite remarkable that no studies proving that ozone is a viable treatment has still been done.

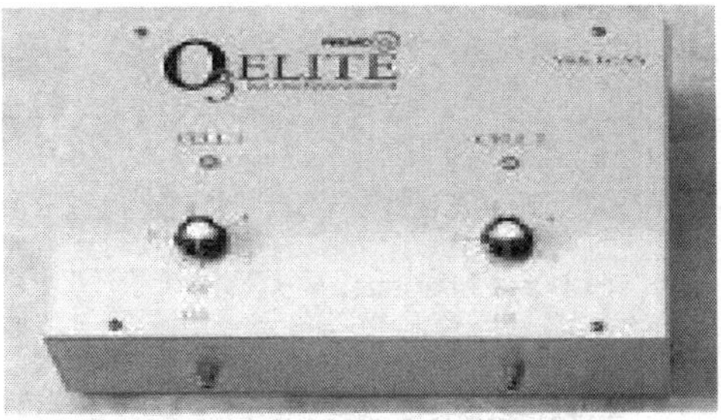

O3 Elite Ozone generator supplied by promolife.com

There are several types of applications the most popular being auto hemoperfusion, funnelling, insufflation, IV, recirculatory hemoperfusion, sauna.

Ozone therapy is used for all conditions and you can get the maximum benefit by applying the right protocol for the right symptom. For example if you are Arthritic then the hand bagging technique may be sufficient. If you have lung cancer then perhaps an ozone sauna with the cupping technique in the sauna would be beneficial. Cancer patients should consider this therapy as the ozone breaks down active oxygen which inturn destroys the cancer cells as cancer cell cannot live in an oxygen rich environment. Ozone also destroys other pathogens and bugs, leaving the rest of the body unharmed.

As the body is cleared of toxins, people who use ozone therapy also report a surge of energy. This therapy can relieve and heal all conditions if applied correctly and depending on your condition coupled with patience, will make you healthy again. Aids, Arthritis, back problems, Candida, Cancers, Carpel tunnel, Lyme and Migraine to name just a few.

There really isn't a down side to this therapy as treatments from practitioners although vary, cost around £50.00 / $100 per session.

Serious life threatening conditions can take up to ten weeks to heal and that could rack up the costs. But buying your own ozone equipment is feasible, around £/$2500, it is a safe protocol with bundles of free information to get you started safely and surely.

Start by reading Ed M^{c}abes' *Flood Your*

Body With Oxygen.

Auto Hemoperfusion

This protocol is used by a small amount of blood via a tube from the vein going into a container with ozone, the ozone cleans the blood which is drained, separating the kill off that the ozone has produced and the clean blood is put back into the body. It is fast and the quickest way to get ozone into the body. To be administered by a physician only.

Recirculatory Hemoperfusion

This protocol takes the blood from one arm, introduces the blood into the ozone chamber (as with Auto hemoperfusion) cleaned and is returned to the body via the other arm. As the name suggests it is not a quick one off drawing of the blood like Auto hemoperfusion, but rather a circulatory process, often used by rock stars to get rid of the highly toxic cocktail of social drugs they consume.

Funnelling

Ozone gas is released from the tube carrying the gas from the ozone generator to a glass cup or funnel which is held over the part of the body where the problem arises. Excellent for the lung, stomach or tissue problems where you want to maximize safe levels of ozone on the problem.

Insufflation

Listed here are a few examples only of the various ozone protocols:

- Ear insufflation is used for ear problems, cranial problems such as migraine or brain tumours and even eye problems.
- Rectal insufflation can be used for colon cleansing, prostate problems or to get the ozone to the stomach area.
- Vaginal insufflation can be used for vaginal conditions, Candida, stomach problems.

IV

Intravenous injections are designed to

achieve the same results as funnelling. The physician will inject ozone directly at the area that is required, in Chile they use this protocol for something as general as a vaccine and for life threatening imbalances such as tumours. Naturally its use is restricted to being administered by a trained professional.

Sauna

Ozone sauna is perhaps the most popular choice as it can be administered at home and used for health maintenance as is for healing. In general the person sits in the sauna for around 20 minutes, in itself is a good thing as this artificially induced hyperthermia raises the body's temperature which kills bacteria and viruses. The sweat glands release toxins helping in the detoxification of the body. Now that the skin pores are open, ozone is applied into the sauna, the ozone has nowhere to go except into the body and after a further short period of time, you simply turn the ozone gas off and have a shower to close the pores so no ozone can escape the body.

Applying this protocol too much too quick may produce a rash, (Herxseimers reaction) as mentioned before, you know then that the protocol is doing its job, and there are supplements you can take to ease or prevent this.

Below are some equally as important Protocols, therapies and natural medicine. **Please do not make the mistake of thinking they are less beneficial that the ones listed previously in greater detail.**

Name	Structure	Description	Benefit
Air Purifier	**Mechanical**	Releases small amounts of ozone into the air.	Best used at the bedside and very beneficial at the hospital bedside for killing bugs after surgery where the body is vulnerable.
Budwig	**Diet**	Cancer and other diseases.	Simply designed to stabilize rather

			than cure – helps if time is short.
Boswellia	**Powder**	A powerful anti-inflammatory.	Arthritis - Brain tumours – Carpel tunnel – Crohn's etc. Shop Boswellia is non effective as they contain additives and low boswellic acids. Visit www.vitalisnews.com for the best quality.
Cellect-Budwig		Stage 4 cancer and other chronic disease including type 2 diabetes.	Rebalances the body You should visit http://www.cellectbudwig.com for full info.
Cesium Chloride	**Ionic Liquid**	A rare metallic chemical element	Raises PH levels making it hard for cancer to thrive.

		used in nuclear medicine.	
Chi Machine	**Mechanical**	Stress buster.	Stimulates muscles and tissues – gently allows the body to absorb more oxygen.
Citricidal	**Liquid**	Anti-microbal.	Grapefruit seed extract – powerful - acts against a large number of pathogenic organisms - bacteria, fungi and viruses.
Colloidal Silver	**Liquid**	Anti-bacterial.	Natures antibiotic –Used regularly can ward off colds and flu's and much more.
Coenzyme C10	**Capsules**	Vital role carrying the source to produce cell energy.	Increase of energy - supports the immune system – assists the

			heart – protects against strokes – destroys free radical and much more.
Crystal therapy	**Solid**	A healing therapy.	Can be used for amongst others symptoms, migraines, digestive and low energy problems.
Dr Batmanhelidj	**Liquid**	Water cure.	Dr Batman has cured many diseases by appropriate use of various quality water.
Dr Coldwell	**Consciousness**	Motivation medicine.	Has cured over 70,00 people some 98% cure rate of cancer by changing though patterns.
Dr Jo Wallach	**Various**	Famed for his book *Dead*	Offers alternative views to once thought

		Doctors Don't Lie.	solid science.
Dr Mercola	**Website**	Excellent resource.	An authority on natural health and medicine.
Dr Simoncini	**IV**	Anti-fungal- used for breast cancer.	Baking soda is injected to the breast neutralizing the fungus – To be administered by a physician only.
Harry Hoxey	**Liquid and Paste**	Removes toxins from the body.	A cancer cure – regarded as a quack in spite of numerous positive testimonies.
Health Science Institute	**Website**	An excellent resource although part of it is subscription.	Offers a lot in the way of first class products but is really geared up to sell, sell, sell. Even so it is still a valuable resource.
MSM	**Crystals,**	An	Enables your

	flakes, powder, tablets, lotion and gel	organic sulphur compound.	cells and tissues to release toxins - Helps repair cellular damage and keeps cell walls permeable, allowing water and nutrients to freely flow.
Natural news	**Website**	Excellent resource.	Pushes the barriers of natural medicine – finding new healthy foods – does tend to bash FDA and CDC etc.
NLP	**Consciousness**	Helps people people understand & organise their thinking & feelings.	Breaks personal patterns of limitations and beliefs - Master your subconscious – master your emotions.
Ozonated Water	**Mechanical**	Water purifier.	Neutralizes pathogens and

			bugs – gives you energy and raises oxygen levels – purifies and cleanses food.
Pinhole Glasses	**Apparatus**	Eye protocol.	A protocol that can restore eyes to 20/20 vision – prevents eye disease.
Royal Raymond Rife	**Mechanical**	Bio resonance.	Neutralizes disease by finding a frequency that destroys the free radical.
SEO	**Liquid**	Oxygen therapy.	Sold as a water purifer this liquid quckly raises your oxygen levels destroying free radical. Used correctly is very powerful.
Jerry Smith	**Author/ protocol**	Pulmonary thrombosis.	Cured himself of the incurable. Visit

			www.jerrysmith.org.
Spiritual Healing	**Energy**	Use of hands to transfer healing energy from a higher source.	People with all conditions go to Spiritual healers.

There many other therapies, protocols and pills readily available, and there are some 600 natural cancer cures, many work better than others. It would take a book of encyclopaedia proportions to list them all and for obvious reasons displaying them would be impractical.

Healing takes place first and foremost with the desire to be whole. The thought, the idea or notion that it is something that you want more than anything else right now at this point in time, a feeling, thrill or emotion embedded deep down inside you is the foundation for healing to take place. Taking responsibility for your own health by verifying the points of interest in this book that concern your immediate problems are the perfect way to start and by doing so, some of the information and references in this book may lead you to seek out a therapy not already detailed, but rather a therapy that may be better suited to your own unique requirements.

As a unique individual you can make that choice and perhaps the hardest decision you will ever make would be to take that first courageous step out of your comfort zone and into the unknown.

Mark Twain wrote: *"Dance like nobody's watching; love like you've never been hurt. Sing like nobody's listening; live like its heaven on earth."*

Right now, this very instant, put down this book and promise yourself a life free of pain and disease. Take that courageous first step, choose life!

Sungazing

"Those who danced were thought to be quite insane by those who could not hear the music."

It was my intention to leave out this section from the book simply because the very the word sungazing or solar gazing

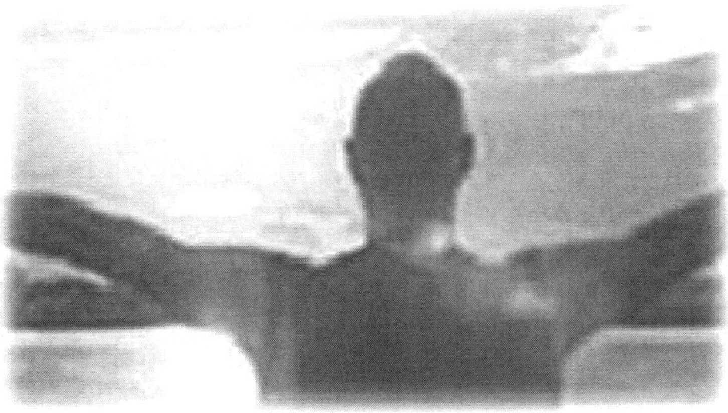

Photograph by Sandy Chase

creates all kinds off fears and biases that society has taught us quite wrongly about this wonderfully simple, natural and yet powerful therapy. But on further consideration I felt that it was far too important to leave out if only because of its simplicity. No training is required, no gurus are required either, you do not have to give up your lifestyle as the sun will correct any imbalances and you will naturally be attracted to what is good for your mind, body, soul development; there is no requirement to stop medication either, as your health improves, your health care practitioner will adjust your medication until no further medicines are required. And one aspect of sungazing we must consider is that this practice is absolutely free.

The sun and her benefits are greatly misunderstood, we have been told only half truths about the sun and the focus of attention has been on how dangerous she is. So before we take a look at sungazing, let's take a short while to add some balance to the sun debate.

Sungazing is not a religion, nor a cult and neither do sungazers worship the sun, we merely look at the sun using a simple protocol to attain, mental, physical and spiritual health.

The education system has taught us that

to look or stare at the sun is harmful and will make you blind, this is a half-truth, if you look at the sun during the midday when the UV rays are high and above two on the UV index then yes, absolutely it will harm your eyes and can sometimes make you blind, for some albeit temporarily.

There is lack of clinical and testimonial information on most historical events simply because looking at the sun has been embedded so deeply in our minds as to be dangerous that there has never truly been open and honest discussion or research, until now! So sungazing is not a new phenomenon, the ancients civilizations of The Aztecs, Egyptians, Mayans, Indian Yogi and many native American Indian tribes to name but a few cultures had been practicing sungazing or many years. Regarded by the man who introduced sungazing to the modern world, *"an old wine in a new bottle"* as he eloquently puts it, HRM or Hira Ratan Manek has reached the pinnacle in the practice of sungazing, and as a consequence has not eaten for years, in fact a documentary was made about him, he was followed and observed for over 411 days by Doctors who did not let him out of their sight and in fact found that he never ate once during this period only taking in some fluid. Of course the purpose of sungazing is not to stop eating; this is merely an option you can choose and once you reach nine months of sungazing hunger will disappear.

It is also believed that the sun will give you skin cancer, again this is another half-truth; if you spend prolonged periods bathing in the sun, then yes, if the conditions in your body are favourable for cancer to develop then there is a real chance that this may happen, but science has also shown that lack of sunlight increases the risk of lung cancer through lack of vitamin D.

Lack of sun produces SAD (Seasonal Affective Disorder). Sweden, a country with very short days in winter has one of the highest suicide rates in Europe. Lack of sunlight promotes Vitamin D

deficiency.
Arthritis is linked to lack of sunshine MS is also linked with lack of sunshine In-fact lack of sunshine promotes disease and healthy sunshine can reverse disease.

There are many examples the naysayers cite when discussing sungazing, almost all of them have made very little or no research at all and as “sheeple” follow the status quo debating and misquoting from arbitrary text, and as a consequence this leads to disempowerment because they do not have to take responsibility for their own health.

So now let’s take a look at the plus side of sungazing and all the benefits the sun offers us. I would firstly like to address the issue of why we must look at the sun as opposed to bathing safely in the sun.

In brief, the eyes are the only part of the body that can receive the entire spectrum of the sunlight. And as we have discussed earlier in this book, your body which functions on a priority basis, will, from the brain distribute the photons of light to which ever part of the body it feels is priority. These photons will also expand your pineal gland regarded by some as the third eye (or the window to the soul) which has been clogged up with chemicals such as Fluoride. The earthly importance of this is that in the winter months when sunshine is few and far between we need our pineal gland functioning correctly as it secretes melatonin, a powerful antioxidant and controller of blood sugar, sleeping and controls pituitary gland, the gland responsible for the body's hormone-producing glands and organs.

The science behind how sungazing heals the body is too vast to discuss fully in this book and nor is it my intention to go into great detail as I want merely to plant the seed of interest and present some facts about sungazing to those of whom it may appeal to.

But I would like to briefly address the issue of cancer and sungazing. Many people have reported to have cured themselves of cancer by adhering to the safe protocols to follow laid out by HRM. Aside from sungazing, cancer patients have also sunbathed during safe sunlight hours for fifteen minutes a day, this practice is best used with minimal clothes and without sun creams which prevent the production of Vitamin D (cancer patients lack vitamin D and sunshine produces vitamin D), they also sunbathe with minimal clothes to allow the full spectrum of light to enter the body through the open pores. HRM also suggests that sungazing and sunbathing is a natural form of chemotherapy, I agree. The sun Oxygenates blood and energizes cells, cancer cells cannot live in an oxygen rich environment! Sungazing also kills bacteria, viruses, and blood-borne pathogens harbouring in your body, and as your body rids itself of diseased cells and pathogens, it has more options to fight remaining diseased cells in the body. Sunbathing is not sufficient, it helps greatly but the real benefit comes from sungazing.

It is worth noting that the practice of sungazing is not *"fast food"* you cannot speed the process up any faster by doing more than the prescribed safe limits neither is anything taken away if you are unable to sungaze for a few days due to weather conditions,; it only slows the rate of progress, you will not have start at the beginning but you can simply continue from where you last left off or reduce your gazing to a more comfortable length of time until your eyes adjust.

There is only so much your body will allow at any one time but you can enhance the process by also walking barefoot on earth or sand. Grass just won't cut it. It is not uncommon to find that the grass you walk barefoot on has been contaminated by chemicals and pesticides and by doing so you will be drawing all those toxins up through your body via your toes. Grass is also known to draw energy from your body! Natural raw earth is better, the sun warms up and energizes the earth allowing barefoot walking full absorption of all the available minerals through the toes, sand by the sea is best, walking on the warm afternoon sand barefoot for 45 minutes is the very best way of harvesting the suns healing energy if no sun available during safe hours.

For those who are still slightly sceptic it is worth noting that walking barefoot activates the pineal gland via the big toe, the remaining four toes also represent glands; the pituitary, (sends signals to other glands and organs), hypothalamus, (responsible for certain metabolic processes and other activities of the autonomic nervous system), thalamus (aids in producing immunity), and amygdala (primary role in the processing of memory and emotional reactions)

So how do we sungaze and for how long, when and where?

For maximum benefit you are better off sungazing barefoot on earth or sand, you could feasibly do this if you have a garden but is not essential. You also have to consider whether or not you can see the sunrise or set from your home. In the winter months if it is too cold to leave the home you can do this by either opening the window while inside the house or if conditions are severe then sungaze with the window closed. For those that live in the city or in a valley you may have to travel hopefully not far to a location where you can sungaze comfortably. Whilst looking at the sun you can blink or flicker your eyes or use pinhole glasses.

Some people also do visualizations, chant, pray, or simply think nice thoughts, while others simply absorb the light, the choice is yours.

If the mind accepts – the body adapts. If the body adapts, the mind accepts! (quote from HRM).

There is one thing we can all do and that is prepare sun charged water, we can drink it, clean our bodies with it and those with myopia or glaucoma who should take great care in this practice can sprinkle this water over their eyes and face. Simply fill a glass jar, the thinner the better, with your favourite water, put a lid on it to prevent anything getting in the container and leave it in the sun from sunrise to sunset, then you can drink the water fully charged with sun energy for up to five hours if you keep it stored in a fridge!

Some people living in very hot countries have been drinking sun charged tea by simply putting water in a cup with their favourite tea and leaving it for a few hours until it's hot and simply drink the sun charged tea!

The protocol and benefits for sungazing safely and effectively are as follows.

Under perfect conditions it should take 9 months of gazing to reach 44 minutes upon which you should not sungaze further but walk barefoot on earth or sand for 45 minutes daily. It is possible also to rather than walk "top up" your energy by sungazing for 15 minutes occasionally, remember each person is individual and must find their own way within the confines of the protocol. You should take off glasses or contact lenses when gazing unless the lens are a fixed part of you person.

You should look at the sun only in the hours of sunrise or sunset, that is to say if the sunrises at 7am, then you can safely gaze between 7am - 8am or if the sunsets at 4pm then you can gaze between 3pm -4pm. These times are when the UV rays on the index are below two and no harm will come to you. The good news is for those in colder climates, in winter, the UV rarely reaches above two and so it is possible to sungaze outside the hours of sunrise and sunset. Regardless of this never, ever gaze during the midday sun hours! You can check the UV index online or most daily newspapers offer this information.

Begin gazing for only 10 seconds at either sunrise or sunset, if 10 seconds is uncomfortable the try five seconds; you could also do five seconds at sunrise and five seconds at sunset. After gazing close your eyes until the sunspots disappear. Now everyday increase the gazing by ten seconds and after three months in a perfect world you should have reached five minutes, during this period which I call the preparatory period, you may notice some changes, nothing to drastic but this will depend on your ability to look out for those little things that no longer happen. Perhaps you may find it easier to get out of bed or your digestion may be slightly better, in my case after only one minute I noticed that my eye floaters where disappearing rapidly, but in the interests of transparency, I had been applying ozone ear insufflation for a while, the results are variable with individuals and it certainly helped my eyes, so in my case the healing process may have started earlier.

Continue increasing the gazing by ten seconds and after three months you would have reached 15 minutes gazing. At this level you start to obtain mental health, confidence and a sense of what is right and wrong. Mental disorders such as Dementia, Alzheimer's, mental depression and other disorders of the brain begin to disappear.

Increasing the gazing 10 seconds daily will once you reach thirty minutes gazing (according to HRM) liberate you of physical disease, and there is plenty of testimony to back this.

Once you have achieved your goal in sungazing you can stop and merely continue with a maintenance program but it is only after thirty five minutes which is around seven and a half months that hunger decreases and your body begins to accept the original form of micro food, which is the sun. Of course the added bonus is that you do not ingest any toxins either with the sun!

Completing the course of 44 minutes will see that you are in perfect health and no need to eat food simply because we do not need food, only energy from the sun that we eat provides the energy. Of course social convention means that there will come a time when visiting friends and family that you may have to eat, but you will not have hunger or desire it.

At this point you must stop sungazing. Forty four minutes is the maximum for the sake of eye health. However if we stop practicing all that good work will get undone and your sun charged body will be discharged so it is essential to continue the practice by walking barefoot on earth or sand for forty five minutes daily. Of course you can after a while continue sungazing for five minutes daily to keep yourself fully charged.

Before sungazing it is essential to have a check-up to make sure that you have no medical problems that the sun could initially make worse, such as glaucoma.

To find out in greater detail about sungazing, its safety and most importantly any safety issues that may be related to you, it is essential to listen to HRM's many lectures. I advise you do not begin sungazing until you listen to his lectures and fully understand the practice.

You can find him on youtube by simply typing in the search box; Sunlight Master at La Casa Day Spa, 41 E 20th NYC HRM Lecture on Sungazing HRM - Sun Gazing - Catalunya (Spain) - 18-April-2009.

Website: http://solarhealing.com

To conclude, I would suggest that you join a sungazing forum if only to keep up to date on how people are progressing and to learn any pitfalls that may have occurred from the over eager gazer.

This therapy promises much and the one aspect of it I can guarantee you is that after the anticipation of waiting for the sunrise or sunset, when you finally start to gaze at the sun you will certainly have a sense of wellness, warmth and great pleasure even after just a couple of minutes of gazing and that alone can only be a positive aspect in our goal for a happy, healthy and enjoyable life.

Remember sungazing costs nothing and if your are seriously ill and have no money to undergo medical treatment, traditional or alternative, then you have nothing to lose by trying this protocol, start by simply accepting the possibility that sungazing may be a solution, do listen to the lectures and join a forum to gain as much information as you can, this protocol does require you to think outside the box, but what do you have to lose!

WEBSITE LINKS

1	**Country of origin** http://www.food.gov.uk/multimedia/pdfs/publication/countryoriginlabellingscot.pdf
2	**Colouring** http://www.food.gov.uk/multimedia/pdfs/guidance.pdf#page=19
3	**Induction of thyroid and liver tumors by chronic exposure to 2-methylimidazole in F344/N rats** and B6C3F1 mice. Chan PC, Sills RC, Kissling GE, Nyska A, Richter W. http://www.ncbi.nlm.nih.gov/pubmed/17924096
4	**Fresh fruit and vegetables** http://www.food.gov.uk/foodindustry/guidancenotes/labelregsguidance/freshpurenaturalguidancenote (31)
5	**Packaging** http://www.food.gov.uk/multimedia/pdfs/fresh.pdf (23/23)
6	**Sulphites** http://www.food.gov.uk/science/research/foodcomponentsresearch/additives/a01programme/a01projlist/a01021/
7	**Adverse reactions to Sulphites** http://www.ncbi.nlm.nih.gov/pmc/articles/PMC1346296/pdf/canmedaj00272-0034.pdf
8	**Dietary intake exposure to sulphites in Italy - analytical determination of sulphite-containing foods and their combination into standard meals for adults and children** C. Leclercqa, M. G. Molinarob, R. Piccinellia, M. Baldinib, D. Arcellaa & P. Stacchinib http://www.tandfonline.com/doi/abs/10.1080/02652030010014402
9	**Cancer risks in hairdressers: Assessment of carcinogenicity of hair dyes and gels** Kamila Czene, Sanna Tiikkaja, Kari Hemminki\ http://onlinelibrary.wiley.com/doi/10.1002/ijc.11040/full

10	**Induction of thyroid and liver tumors by chronic exposure to 2-methylimidazole in F344/N rats and B6C3F1 mice.** Chan PC, Sills RC, Kissling GE, Nyska A, Richter W. http://www.ncbi.nlm.nih.gov/pubmed/17924096
11	**Toxicity and carcinogenicity studies of 4-methylimidazole in F344/N rats and B6C3F1 mice** P. C. Chan, R. C. Sills, G. E. Kissling, A. Nyska and W. Richter http://www.springerlink.com/content/?Author=G.+E.+Kissling
12	**Consumption of Soft Drinks With Phosphoric Acid As a Risk Factor for the Development of Hypocalcemia in Postmenopausal Women** Guerrero-Romero Fernando Rodriguez-Moran Martha Reyes Evangelina http://www.jclinepi.com/article/S0895-4356(99)00097-9/abstract
13	**Caffeine In Colas: "The Real Thing" Isn't The Taste** http://esgweb1.nts.jhu.edu/press/2000/AUGUST/000814.HTM
14	**Trans Fatty Acids and Cardiovascular Disease** Mozaffarian, Dariush; Katan, Martijn B.; Ascherio, Alberto; Stampfer, Meir J.; Willett, Walter C. http://journals.lww.com/obgynsurvey/Abstract/2006/08000/Trans_Fatty_Acids_and_Cardiovascular_Disease.20.aspx
15	**Meat intake, heterocyclic amines, and risk of breast cancer: a case-control study in Uruguay.** E De Stefani, A Ronco, M Mendilaharsu, M Guidobono and H Deneo-Pellegrini http://cebp.aacrjournals.org/content/6/8/573.short
16	**Cancer risk of heterocyclic amines in cooked foods: an analysis and implications for research** David W. Layton, Kenneth T. Bogen, Mark G. Knize1, Fred T. Hatch1, Virginia M. Johnson and James S. Felton http://carcin.oxfordjournals.org/content/16/1/39.short

17	**Meat intake and bladder cancer risk in 2 prospective cohort studies.** Michaud DS, Holick CN, Giovannucci E, Stampfer MJ. http://www.ncbi.nlm.nih.gov/pubmed/17093172
18	**Diet and pancreatic cancer: a case-control study** STAFFAN E. NORELL ANDERS AHLBOM ROLF ERWALD GőRAN JACOBSON3 INGER LINDBERG-NAVIER ROBERT OLIN BO TőRNBERG and KARL-LUDVIG WIECHEL http://aje.oxfordjournals.org/content/124/6/894.short
19	**food chart for salt content** http://healthyeatingclub.com/info/books-phds/books/foodfacts/html/data/data5a.html
20	**Reductive stress linked to heart disease -University of Utah Health Sciences** http://www.eurekalert.org/pub_releases/2007-08/uouh-rsl080707.php
21	**Cigarette, alcohol, and caffeine consumption: risk factors for spontaneous abortion** **Vibeke Rasch** http://onlinelibrary.wiley.com/doi/10.1034/j.1600-0412.2003.00078.x/full
22	**Alcohol Consumption and Alcoholic Liver Disease: Evidence of a Threshold Level of Effects of Ethanol** V. T. Savolainen K. Liesto A. Männikkö A. Penttilä P. J. Karhunen http://onlinelibrary.wiley.com/doi/10.1111/j.1530-0277.1993.tb05673.x/abstract
23	**Formaldehyde Exposure among Industrial Workers Is Associated with Increased Risk of Cancers of the Blood and Lymphatic System** http://www.cancer.gov/newscenter/pressreleases/2009/formaldehyde
24	**First Experimental Demonstration of the Multipotential Carcinogenic Effects of Aspartame Administered in the Feed to Sprague-Dawley Rats**

	Morando Soffritti, Fiorella Belpoggi, Davide Degli Esposti, Luca Lambertini, Eva Tibaldi, and Anna Rigano http://www.ncbi.nlm.nih.gov/pmc/articles/PMC1392232/
25	**Increasing Brain Tumor Rates: Is There a Link to Aspartame?** Oney, John W. MD; Farber, Nuri B.; Spitznagel, Edward; Robins, Lee N. http://journals.lww.com/jneuropath/Abstract/1996/11000/Increasing_Brain_Tumor_Rates__Is_There_a_Link_to.2.aspx
26	**Aspartame as a Dietary Trigger of Headache** Richard B. Lipton M.D.1,2, Lawrence C. Newman M.D.1, Joel S. Cohen M.D.1, Seymour Solomon M.D.1,2 http://onlinelibrary.wiley.com/doi/10.1111/j.1526-4610.1989.hed2902090.x/abstract
27	**An earlier age of breast cancer diagnosis related to more frequent use of antiperspirants/deodorants and underarm shaving.** McGrath KG. http://www.ncbi.nlm.nih.gov/pubmed/14639125?itool=EntrezSystem2.PEntrez.Pubmed.Pubmed_ResultsPanel.Pubmed_RVDocSum&ordinalpos=3
28	**Carcinogenicity of the Drinking Water Mutagen 3-Chloro-4-(dichloromethyl)-5-hydroxy-2(5H)-furanone in the Rat** Hannu Komulainen, Sirkka-Liisa Vaittinen, Terttu Vartiainen and Jouko Tuomisto http://jnci.oxfordjournals.org/content/89/12/848.short
29	**Trihalomethanes and associated potential cancer risks in the water supply in Ankara, Turkey.** Tokmak B, Capar G, Dilek FB, Yetis U. **http://www.ncbi.nlm.nih.gov/pubmed/15364603**
30	**Opinion of the Scientific Panel on Dietetic Products, Nutrition and Allergies (NDA) on a request from the Commission related to the Tolerable Upper Intake Level of Fluoride**

	http://www.efsa.europa.eu/en/efsajournal/pub/192.htm
31	**The International Chemical Safety Cards** http://www.cdc.gov/niosh/ipcs/icstart.html
32	**Fluoride, an essential nutrient.** http://www.nap.edu/openbook.php?record_id=2204&page=30
33	**Fluoride water 'causes cancer' Boys at risk from bone tumours, shock research reveals** http://www.guardian.co.uk/society/2005/jun/12/medicineandhealth.genderissues
34	**Health Canada** http://www.fluoridealert.org/canada.2009.report.pdf
35	**Bfs website** http://www.bfsweb.org/facts/tech_aspects/chem.htm
36	**What the problem is.** http://www.whattheproblemis.com/documents/mot/mot_Biological_Effects_of_Fluorides.pdf
37	**Healthy communications** http://www.healthy-communications.com/expertsapologyonfluoride.html
38	**Toxicological overview** http://www.hpa.org.uk/webc/HPAwebFile/HPAweb_C/1227169969666
39	**Journal of the American College of Toxicology** http://www.healthy-communications.com/slsalert.html
40	**Final Report on the Safety Assessment of Sodium Lauryl Sulfate and Ammonium Lauryl Sulfate** http://ijt.sagepub.com/content/2/7/127
41	**Diseases of modern living: neurological changes associated with mobile phones and radiofrequency radiation in humans** Roderick Westerman Bruce Hocking http://www.sciencedirect.com/science/article/pii/S0304394003014149
42	**Mobile phone From Wikipedia** http://en.wikipedia.org/wiki/Mobile_phone

43	http://jimhumble.biz http://genesis2church.org
44	http://mmsnews.org
45	http://www.genesis2forum.org/index.php?option=com_kunena&view=entrypage&defaultmenu=68&Itemid=66
46	http://www.glycaemicindex.com/